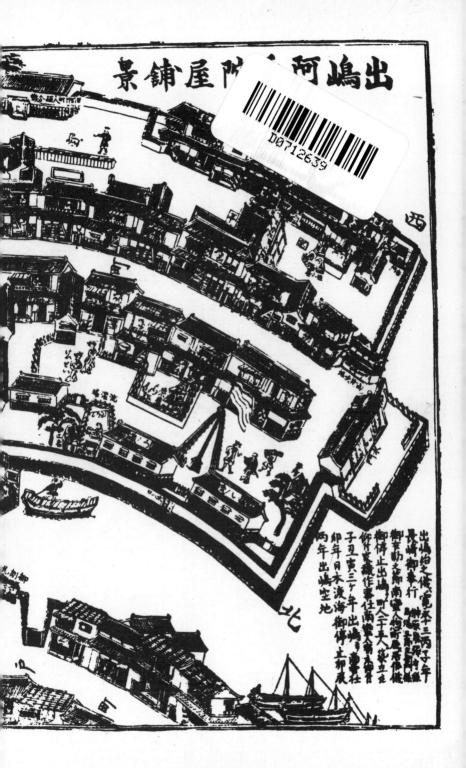

景鋪屋陀蘭阿嶋出

西

北

出嶋伯之儀、寛永十三丙子年長崎御奉行
御建勅之御南蛮人の新堂居催
御傳止出嶋、町人三十大家三十
竹作家藪仕南蛮人新堂石の
子丑寅三ヶ年出嶋御傳止御辰
卯年日本渡海御傳止御辰
両年出嶋空地

Western Medical Pioneers
in Feudal Japan

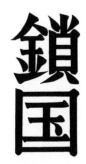

Western Medical Pioneers
in Feudal Japan

John Z. Bowers

Published for
The Josiah Macy, Jr. Foundation
by
The Johns Hopkins Press
Baltimore and London

End Papers: A woodcut of the Dutch
settlement at Deshima, Nagasaki,
by Toshimaya Bunjiuemon. From
N. H. N. Mody, *A Collection of
Nagasaki Colour Prints and
Paintings* . . . (Rutland, Vt.:
Charles E. Tuttle Co., 1969).

The Johns Hopkins Press, Baltimore, Maryland 21218
The Johns Hopkins Press Ltd., London

Library of Congress Catalog Card Number 73-86098

Standard Book Number 8018-1081-7

I dedicate this book to my parents, Adelaide and John, who made many sacrifices so that I might study medicine.

Contents

The characters on the case and title page read *sakou*, "closed country," the term the Japanese applied to their country during the two centuries described in this book. The calligraphy on the case, title page, and chapter openings was drawn by Mr. Isamu Kawai.

I Medicine man: A Japanese doctor on his way to visit a patient, followed by an attendant who carries a traveling case containing instruments. Drawn by Keisai Kugawata in the middle of the Edo period (1616-1867). Courtesy of CIBA SYMPOSIA, formerly published by CIBA Pharmaceutical Company, Summit, New Jersey.

II Hollander: The Dutch feasting at Deshima, attended by their Javanese servants. From N. H. N. Mody, *A Collection of Nagasaki Colour Prints and Paintings* . . . (Rutland, Vt.: Charles E. Tuttle Co., 1969).

III *Opperhoofd*: An *opperhoofd* and his Javanese slave, ca. 1780. From the original in the General J. C. Pabst collection of C. R. Boxer, reproduced in his book *Jan Compagnie in Japan, 1600-1850*, 2d rev. ed. (The Hague: Martinus Nijhoff, 1950).

IV *Schellach*: A Nagasaki woodcut of the Dutch East India ship *Schellach*. From the original formerly in the collection of C. R. Boxer, reproduced in his book *Jan Compagnie in Japan, 1600-1850*, 2d rev. ed. (The Hague: Martinus Nijhoff, 1950).

V Porch scene, Nagasaki: A Hollander dividing his attention between a geisha and sake, yet watching Deshima. Note that a European-style chandelier has been transplanted to the geisha house. From the author's collection.

VI The Nihon-bashi Bridge, by Yasuda Raishū. From *Pictorial Record of Kobe City Museum of Nanban Art*. Courtesy of Kobe Municipal Art Museum of Nanban, Japan.

Introduction

Medicine was the key force in the development of Western knowledge in Japan during the two centuries when that country was "closed" to the West. When Commodore Matthew Perry arrived in Japanese waters in 1853, Japanese physicians had been practicing Western medicine in Nagasaki, Osaka, Kyoto, and Edo (now Tokyo) for eighty years. The translation in 1774 of a German anatomy text into Japanese by Japanese was in some respects an event as significant in the rise of Western influences in Japan as the arrival of the Commodore.

For two centuries beginning in 1641, the only Japanese contact with the West was through a Dutch trading post on the small island of Deshima in Nagasaki Bay. There was usually a European doctor on the staff, and from the beginning the doctors taught Dutch, Western medicine, and natural history to the Japanese. These doctors ranged in ability from barber-surgeons to four remarkable physician-explorers—a Hollander, a Swede, and two Germans.

Of at least equal significance was the singular concern of the Japanese for medicine and health, a cultural trait which has impressed many visitors through the centuries. This unique interest in medicine brought the Japanese to Nagasaki to study with the European doctors and to question them night and day about medicine when they visited Kyoto and Edo on their journey to report to the military ruler on the state of the world.

Thus an abiding interest in medicine and health and the presence of European doctors at Nagasaki were leading forces in the westernization of Japan. In 1870, two years after the overthrow of the isolationist military rulers and the enthronement of the Emperor Meiji, Japan made the wise decision to adopt German medicine, and twelve students were sent to Germany for training.

From September, 1962, until June, 1964, I was a Visiting Professor at Kyoto National University. Soon after I had established myself in the most comfortable office I have ever known, Japanese medical students began to knock on my door seeking an opportunity to practice English, which in turn afforded me an opportunity to learn about Japan. Japanese professors began to tell me with remarkable candor about their programs and problems, and I was launched on a full-scale study of medical education in Japan.

As I listened to the Japanese professors talk about their systems of medical education, strange names—Deshima, *Oranda*, Kaempfer, Thunberg, and Siebold were repeated. I decided that my book about medical education should begin with a few chapters tracing the development of Western medicine in Japan. In 1965 this study was published under the title *Medical Education in Japan.*

A number of people who read that book said the most interesting chapters pertained to the island of Deshima. I had already become fascinated with the Deshima story and had begun to gather material for a complete study of the rise of Western medicine in Japan.

The study led to many expeditions abroad to gather information on the explorers who had served at Deshima. These journeys took me to Lemgo, Detmold, the British Museum, and the Museum for Natural History for Kaempfer; Uppsala and Paris for Thunberg; Bonn, Munich, Würzburg, The Hague, and Leiden for Siebold. The final visit was to Schloss Mittelbiberach in Swabia, Germany, where I was the overnight guest of Siebold's great-grandson, Alexander, Graf von Brandenstein-Zeppelin. He gave me the opportunity to inspect many important documents on Siebold. At Leiden I received invaluable support from Dr. Cornelius Ouwehand, and at Bonn, from an old friend, Professor Johannes Steudel.

The first book that I read relating to Western medicine in Japan was *Jan Compagnie in Japan*, one of the many excellent manuscripts of Professor Charles R. Boxer. It was a significant factor in my beginning the studies that led to the present book. Subsequently, I have had the good fortune to establish a close relationship with Charles Boxer, and he has spent many hours working with me and encouraging me to get on with my studies.

My principal teachers in Japan have been Professors Teizo Ogawa of Juntendo University and Ranzaburō Ōtori of Keio University. Professor Michio Okamoto at Kyoto University uncovered a wealth of material in the Fujikawa collections. Professor Jirō Numata made available important sources on the period of *Rangaku*. Professor Teizo Ogawa and Professor Boxer have read this manuscript and I am deeply grateful for their comments and corrections.

Miss Mayumi Taniguchi, Mrs. Atsumi Minami, and Mrs. Teruko Kusama have spent many hours working with Japanese sources on my behalf. Mr. Yoshinari Tsuda, librarian at Keio, assisted in the procurement of materials.

Mrs. Catherine L. Coughlin, Mr. Hubert W. Mullings, and Miss Phyllis M. Brachman were invaluable associates in the preparation of the final manuscript and the assembly of the illustrations. Miss Helen Choat gave important advice on the organization of the material.

A final concentrated burst of effort to complete this manuscript was made possible by a generous invitation from The Rockefeller Foundation to spend the month of July, 1968, in residence at Villa Serbelloni on Lake Como, Italy.

Finally, I am specially indebted to the directors of the Macy Foundation, who have tolerated, without complaint, my travels and my commitment to Japanese studies.

JOHN Z. BOWERS, M.D.

Western Medical Pioneers
in Feudal Japan

壱

CHAPTER

I

Medicine before the Dutch

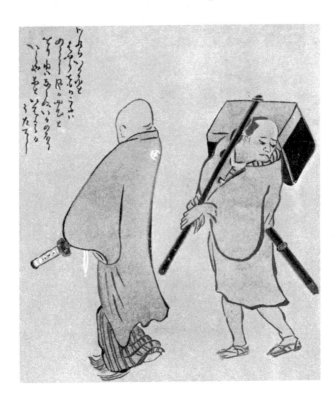

As the visitor to Nagasaki today walks westward from the heart of the city, he descends a hill, reaches a canal, and observes on the far bank a small, fenced garden. The garden is a memorial on the site of the historic island of Deshima where for more than two centuries a handful of Hollanders under strict guard maintained the only remnants of a century of Western approaches to Japan. After the almost total exclusion of the outside world from Japan in 1641, for reasons of trade and status the Dutch chose to remain on Deshima and to live under the most prison-like conditions ever willingly endured by free men. Yet, despite all obstacles, an exchange of information on Western and oriental culture, especially with regard to medicine, continued between the Dutch and the Japanese. The principal figures in this exchange were physicians, and the principal interest of the Japanese who came to Deshima was Western medicine. Thus medicine was the key field that brought Western knowledge to Japan more than two centuries before Perry "opened" the empire to the West in 1853.

The abundant plants and shrubs in the Deshima garden and an arbor inside the gate remind the visitor that three centuries ago European doctors began to cultivate Japanese plants there for subsequent transfer to the gardens of Europe. An old cannon from an East Indiaman that foundered in a typhoon recalls that the greatest of these doctors, Philipp von Siebold, was expelled from Japan. One reason was that his foundering ship revealed a treasure trove of forbidden Japanese materials presented to him by grateful Japanese students. In a shaded corner an oval stone just a few feet high bears the inscription "*Ecce virent vestrae hic plantae florentque quotannis. Cultorum memores serta feruntque pia*" ("Look how your plants are flourishing and blossoming every year, remembering their cultivators and bearing pious garlands"). These lines memorialize the three leading European doctors who served at Deshima—Engelbert Kaempfer, Carl Pieter Thunberg, and Philipp von Siebold, who struck the inscription in the 1820's to commemorate these his most illustrious predecessors.

Beside the garden is a warehouse restored along sturdy Dutch lines, and in the dark and dusty center of the next building may be seen old beams left by the Dutch, bearing insignia in Latin.

On the street corner is a classical Dutch-style building of the Deshima period.

When the Dutch were locked behind the walls of Deshima in 1641, Chinese traditional medicine, *Chung-i*, which the Japanese called *Kampō*, was the system of medicine then followed in Japan. It was practically unknown in the West.

Before the introduction of *Chung-i*, medicine in Japan was indigenous and emphasized a close association between health and disease and the native religion, Shinto. The major sources on this indigenous medicine are two semimythical chronicles: the *Nihon Shoki* [Chronicles of Japan], A.D. 720, and the *Kojiki* [Chronicles of ancient times], A.D. 712. They attribute the origins of medicine to two semideities, Ō-na-muchi-no-mikoto and Sukuna-hikona-no-mikoto. The sick received charms and amulets from the priests, and medications were primarily natural products —powdered clamshell in sea water for burns and cattails mixed with animal fat for wounds. Baths in hot mineral springs were recommended for a wide range of disorders.

Korea, where Chinese culture was firmly implanted, served for several centuries as the cultural bridge between China and Japan. The first practitioner of *Chung-i* to visit Japan, Kon Mu, was sent by the king of Silla, a kingdom in southeast Korea, in A.D. 414 at the request of the emperor, Inkyō Tennō, who was unable to walk. Soon after, a group of scholars, including physicians, was sent across by the ruler of another Korean kindgom, Paekche, as an offering of thanks for the military protection that the kingdom was receiving from Japan. A century later, in A.D. 552, a major Korean delegation representing Chinese culture came to Japan, bringing musicians, artists, and Confucian scholars, as well as medical practitioners and herbalists. Their gifts included Chinese texts on medicine: *Nan-kyo*, on difficult diseases; *Reisu*, on internal medicine; and *Sho-hin*, on miscellaneous prescriptions.

The first Korean visitor described as a teacher of medicine was Kwan Roku, who taught *Chung-i* to twenty young men nominated by the imperial court at the beginning of the seventh century. In a few years the Japanese established a direct bridge with China, and this coincided with the emergence of the magnificent T'ang dynasty. This regime rapidly took China to the position of the

3

richest, most powerful, most opulent, and best-governed country in the world. It was only natural that the island-isolated Japanese should turn to China as the great storehouse of culture, and there followed a massive flow of Confucian philosophy, Buddhism, painting, pottery, language, and medicine—perhaps every aspect of the Chinese way of life save one of its greatest contributions, the Chinese cuisine—into Japan.

Chung-i

Chinese traditional medicine continued to be the basis of the Japanese system of medicine for many centuries. The origins of Chinese traditional medicine relate to the dawn of Chinese civilization; the complete systemization and spread of *Chung-i* throughout the empire occurred during the Han dynasty, from 202 B.C. to A.D. 220. *Chung-i* is based on the belief that the individual is a microcosm in the larger universe, which is constantly interacting with and influencing his body and all of his activities. Health is dependent upon the maintenance of "harmony" in a highly complex series of relationships. There is a central unity, *Tao*, the "Way," and everywhere, the human body included, there are two opposing forces which must be maintained in perfect balance: *yang* is male—bright, warm, and positive—while *yin* is female—dark, cold, and negative. There are five basic elements—wood, water, earth, fire, and metal—from which spring a variety of relationships, including the organs of the body, seasons, colors, tastes, and symbols. Thus the relationships of wood include the liver, the eyes, the ligaments, springtime, anger, tears, wind, sour, green, charity, Jupiter, morning, green dragon (representing the emperor), and east. The five parenchymatous organs—liver, kidneys, heart, lungs, and spleen—are *yin* organs while the hollow structures—stomach, gall bladder, bladder, small intestine, and large intestine—are *yang* organs. There are three "warmers" or "burning spaces" for the thorax, upper abdomen, and lower abdomen respectively. Between the kidneys is a structure called the "Gate of Life," and there are five throats. The Chinese held the human body in such awe that they considered it a profound sacrilege to damage it, and there were few efforts at dissection or surgery.

4

The diagnosis of disease according to *Chung-i* is based primarily upon meticulous palpation of the pulse at each wrist. There are three major segments at each wrist representing specific organs, and these in turn are subdivided into seven superficial or *liao* pulses and eight deep or *li* pulses. The practitioner is concerned not only with the rate but also with the strength and direction of the beat. Observation of the tongue for color, furring, vascularity, and moisture is a second diagnostic maneuver, and the third is an assessment of the general attitude of the patient. The patient's attitude is especially important because of the emphasis placed on the relationship between particular emotions—gladness, shock, fear, sadness, contemplation, worry, anger—and disease.

As there is a triad of diagnostic approaches, so there is a therapeutic triad—medicines, acupuncture, and moxibustion. The Chinese developed a truly enormous materia medica in which the two principal therapeutic agents are the forked root, or ginseng, and powdered horn or antler. Medicines are frequently prescribed in mixtures of ten or more ingredients.

The therapeutic technique of *Chung-i* which has achieved the greatest notoriety is acupuncture. Its use is based on the belief that within the body there are six basic meridians or channels of *yang* and six of *yin*. From these springs an intricate network of subsidiary channels which connects the organs with 365 points on the skin. For each organ there are a number of skin points scattered across the body, and through the insertion of slender needles into the appropriate skin points the disorder in an organ will be alleviated.

The basis for the use of moxibustion in the treatment of disease is the same as that for acupuncture. The dried leaves of the mugwort (*Artemisia vulgaris*) are rolled into small pellets, ignited, and applied to the skin points until redness and blistering develop.

The Japanese placed greater emphasis on moxibustion than on acupuncture and applied the burning cones to themselves and to each other without the services of a practitioner. Similarly, they indulged in far more self-medication than did the Chinese, in part because of their striking sensitivity to minor deviations from a complete sense of well-being and their deep faith in medicine.

The introduction of Buddhism from China in the sixth century also was significant for medicine in Japan. The priests combined their religious teachings with an emphasis on the healing powers of the sutras, and the first charitable institutions that they established included infirmaries. Disease played a decisive role in the official adoption of Buddhism by the court when Emperor Yōmei became a Buddhist in the vain hope that his new religious affiliation would cure a fatal illness.

In A.D. 702 the Taihō ("Great Treasure") Code of Laws, which was modeled after the Chinese system, was promulgated. It called for a comprehensive educational program marked by the establishment of a *daigaku* ("university") in the capital city of Nara and *kokugaku* ("provincial schools") in each of the provinces, all of which included education in medicine. However, only the sons of the nobility and high-ranking court officials were admitted. Thus, as Sir George Sansom has emphasized: "The Japanese failed, in borrowing the greatest of all Chinese institutions, to take over its essence, which was a respect for learning coupled with a desire for its spread. They seem to have refrained very deliberately from tampering with the aristocratic structure of their own society, and we may here fitly anticipate by stating that in the long run they paid a heavy price for this neglect" (Sansom, 1952, p. 112).

The Taihō Code proposed that medicine should be a profession restricted to the privileged classes, with six categories of students: *i-sei* ("medical student"), *anma-sei* ("massage student"), *shin-sei* ("acupuncture student"), *jo-i-sei* ("student for diseases of women"), *yaku-en-sei* ("pharmacy student"), and *zukkin-sei* ("elective student"). All students would study Chinese medical literature as well as *Ko-Kiyo* [The book of filial piety] and *Rongo* [The Confucian analects]. The study of internal medicine, diseases of women, or acupuncture called for a program of seven years; pediatrics or surgery, five years; and massage or shampooing, three years.

The formidable Chinese examination system was included in the program, and a candidate for medicine would take a monthly examination before the faculty, an annual examination before the chief medical officer of the province, and the final examination before the Chief Minister of the Imperial Court.

Because of a total lack of national unity and constant and bitter civil war, the program set forth in the Taihō Code was never launched. A short-lived *daigaku* was established in the capital city some twenty years after the enunciation of the code. Physicians continued to be trained as apprentices, and their sons traditionally followed unquestioningly in their footsteps. Medical care was, in general, restricted to the families of rank. A hospital was established in the capital city of Nara in A.D. 730, and the first official record of a smallpox epidemic was inscribed in 735.

Recurrent epidemics in the latter part of the eighth century took the lives of thousands of people and shook the faith of the emperor in the medicine from China and in the role of the Buddhist priests as physicians. He tried briefly to revive Japanese indigenous medicine but soon returned to *Kampō*.

The most detailed descriptions of the practices of *Kampō* are contained in the *Ishinho*, which is probably the oldest medical book written in Japan that is available today. Totaling thirty volumes, *Ishinho* was completed by a Japanese physician, Tamba Yasuyori, in A.D. 982–84. There were innumerable indications for the use of acupuncture and of moxibustion. Skin infections were prevalent in Japan and moxibustion was considered to be beneficial for abscesses. When drainage had been accomplished, washing with a solution of crushed rose petals and coptis roots, followed by rubbing with fat of the wild boar, was recommended. Horns were held to have unlimited value, and powdered antler kneaded with hollyhock seeds and applied as a poultice would cause the prompt disappearance of an infection.

To allay pain a cooled stone or iron, or a paste of millet powder mixed in the white of an egg, was recommended. Particulate substances, including lime, white ashes, powdered oyster shell, and gypsum, were applied to the site of a hemorrhage.

With the fall of the T'ang dynasty early in the tenth century, Japan moved toward greater self-sufficiency in all fields, but Chinese traditional medicine continued to be the basis for Japanese medicine. The almost incessant wars attracted the best youth to bear arms or to enter administrative posts. The practitioners of medicine were predominantly individuals who for physical or mental reasons were not qualified for military service.

A different approach to disease as embodied in the *Ritokan* and *Shutankei*, commonly known as the *Ri-shū* school, was introduced from China by Tashiro Sanki, also known as Dodo (1465–1537). The *Ri-shū* system emphasized that disease could be caused by factors other than the cosmic imbalances that were the basis of traditional *Kampō*.

Tashiro's leading student was a Kyoto youth, Manase Dōsan (1507–94), and he was responsible for the dissemination of *Ri-shū* in central and southern Japan.

After twelve years in the study of Buddhism at Kyoto, Manase, a highly dedicated student, entered the study of Chinese ethics and history at the Ashikaga-gakkō, northwest of Tokyo, at this period Japan's leading educational center. It was established at about the time of the Taihō Code, in 702, and in Manase Dōsan's years was probably the sole surviving institution of that ambitious program. Its reputation was based largely on the patronage of the Uyesugi family, which acquired many classical books from China for the school's library.

Three years later Manase began to study medicine under Tashiro Sanki and in 1545, after thirteen years with Tashiro, he returned to Kyoto. Here he established a school, Keiteki-in, where he taught both medicine and Confucian analects. He collected many of the old Japanese medical texts and published their theories of medicine in an eight-volume text, *Keiteki-shū*, in 1574. For diagnosis Manase emphasized observation of the urine, at that time an essential diagnostic feature of medical practice in Europe. He was a court favorite because of his medical skill and his scholarship, and when he presented a copy of his book to the mikado he was rewarded with the honorific title *suichiku-in* ("green bamboo garden").

The practitioners of the *Ri-shū* school drew up a set of rules for their students which emphasized the priestly role of the physician and the secrecy with which medical practices were guarded in Japan in the sixteenth century:

THE 17 RULES OF ENJUIN
(FOR DISCIPLES IN OUR SCHOOL)

1. Each person should follow the path designated by Heaven (Buddha, the Gods).

2. You should always be kind to people. You should always be devoted to loving people.

3. The teaching of Medicine should be restricted to selected persons.

4. You should not tell others what you are taught, regarding treatments, without permission.

5. You should not establish association with doctors who do not belong to this school.

6. All the successors and descendants of the disciples of this school shall follow the teachers' ways.

7. If any disciples cease the practice of Medicine, or, if successors are not found at the death of the disciple, all the medical books of this school should be returned to the SCHOOL OF ENJUIN.

8. You should not kill living creatures, nor should you admire hunting or fishing.

9. In our school, teaching about poisons is prohibited, nor should you receive instructions about poisons from other physicians. Moreover, you should not give abortives to the people.

10. You should rescue even such patients as you dislike or hate. You should do virtuous acts, but in such a way that they do not become known to people. To do good deeds secretly is a mark of virtue.

11. You should not exhibit avarice and you must not strain to become famous. You should not rebuke or reprove a patient, even if he does not present you with money or goods in gratitude.

12. You should be delighted, if, after treating a patient without success, the patient receives medicine from another physician, and is cured.

13. You should not speak ill of other physicians.

14. You should not tell what you have learned from the time you enter a woman's room, and, moreover, you should not have obscene or immoral feelings when examining a woman.

15. Proper or not, you should not tell others what you have learned in lectures, or what you have learned about prescribing medicine.

16. You should not like undue extravagance. If you like such living, your avarice will increase, and you will lose the ability to be kind to others.

17. If you do not keep the rules and regulations of this school, then you will be cancelled as a disciple. In more severe cases, the punishment will be greater.*

The first Europeans to reach Japan were the Portuguese in 1542. There followed a century of contact with the Portuguese and later the Spaniards in which trade and Christian missions were the principal aims of the Iberians. With the Portuguese missions came the Jesuits; intelligent, courageous, militant, and uncompromising, they concentrated their efforts on the upper classes and in general followed the Jesuit policy of only limited medical programs. In their missionary efforts they were uniquely successful, and by the beginning of the seventeenth century there were 300,000 converts in a country of 15 million people.

It was customary for the Jesuits to prepare frequent detailed reports for headquarters at Goa, and one of these, by Father Luis Frois, describes the contrasting practices of Western and Japanese medicine in the middle of the sixteenth century:

1. Amongst us, scrofula, pain from stone, gout and bubonic plague are frequent things; all of these diseases are rare in Japan.

2. We use bleeding; the Japanese, buttons of fire with herbs.

3. The men amongst us are accustomed ordinarily to bleed from the arms; the Japanese with leeches or with a knife on the forehead, and the horses with a lancet.

4. We use clysters or syringes; they in no case use this remedy.

5. Amongst us the physicians prescribe through pharmacies; the Japanese physicians send the medicines from their houses.

6. Our physicians take the pulse of men and of women first on the right arm, afterwards on the left; the Japanese, for men, first on the left and for women, first on the right.

7. Our physicians look at the urine in order to have more information of the illness; the Japanese in no case look at it.

8. The flesh of Europeans, through being delicate, heals very slowly; that of the Japanese, through being robust, heals much better and more quickly from severe wounds, abrasions, infections and accidents.

* William O. Reinhardt provided me with this translation by personal communication in 1962.

9. Amongst us wounds are sutured; the Japanese place on them a little adhesive paper.

10. We make all bandages with cloth; the Japanese make them with paper.

11. Amongst us all abscesses are burnt with fire; the Japanese will die before using our harsh surgical remedies.

12. If our sick are fasting, one works to force them to eat; the Japanese consider this cruel and if the sick are fasting, they thus let them die.

13. Our sick are in cots or beds with sheets, mattresses and pillows; the Japanese upon a board on the floor with a block of wood and their kimono as cover.

14. In Europe one has hens and chickens as medicine for the sick; the Japanese consider this poisonous and order to give them fish and salted turnip.

15. We extract teeth with pincers, tooth forceps, pliers, etc.; the Japanese with chisel and mallet, or with a bow and arrow tied to the tooth, or with blacksmith's tongs.

16. Our spices and medicines are ground in a mortar; in Japan they are ground in a boat-shaped dish of copper with a wheel of iron held between the hands.

17. Amongst us pearls are used for personal ornamentation; in Japan they serve for nothing more than to be ground to make medicines.

18. Amongst us, if a physician is not examined, there is a penalty and he cannot practice; in Japan, in order to make a living, whoever wants to can be a physician.

19. Amongst us for a man to become ill with a venereal disease is always a filthy and shameful thing; the Japanese men and women consider this a common thing and take no shame for it [translated from Frois, 1585, pp. 206–11].

The first practitioner of Western medicine in Japan was a Portuguese, Luis d'Almeida, a successful trader who became a devoted medical missionary in the Society of Jesus and a philanthropist. Under the fires of the Inquisition his Jewish family had apostasized. He himself joined the society in Japan and financed its Japanese programs with money that he had gained while

11

trading between Malacca, Siam, and China in league with a one-eyed Portuguese sailor-adventurer, Duarte da Gama.

Almeida was born in Lisbon about 1525 and studied surgery at the famed Real de Todos-os-Santos Hospital in Lisbon. This venerable institution was established under a papal bull by King John II in 1498 as a merger of thirty-eight small hospitals of religious orders in Lisbon. It was designed in the shape of a cross with an entry wing and three patient-care units. One wing, St. Vincent's, was for infectious diseases; the second, St. Cosmos, for wounds; and the third, Santa Clara, for female patients. Beneath the four wings was a series of colonnades that served as homes for the poor. At the end of each of the three clinical wings there was a pool of water for cleansing the sick and their garments.

The students at Todos-os-Santos usually enrolled in a two-year apprentice system after which they were permitted to practice as second-level doctors. At the end of their apprenticeship they were examined in medicine by the *fisico-mor* ("chief physician") and in surgery by the *cirugiao-mor* ("chief surgeon"), who were nominated as heads of their respective professions by the crown. Luis d'Almeida received his certificate in March, 1546.

To satisfy his thirst for adventure, Almeida sailed for the Indies about 1548 and fell in with Duarte da Gama, who had lost an eye and several fingers in a sea battle and had been imprisoned for the pillage of a pagoda near Quilon in Malabar.

Almeida and da Gama's first trading voyage was to Sanchan (Chang-tch'ouan, also Chang-chuan), a barren island about thirty leagues off Canton where Portuguese merchants had been secretly trading for twenty years. They then visited two Japanese ports frequented by Portuguese traders: Hirado Island in Hizen Province and Funai in Bungo. The lords of both fiefs, especially the lord of Hizen, actively solicited trade with the Portuguese.

At Hirado Island, Almeida and da Gama found the great Jesuit missionary Francis Xavier and his two companions, Cosme de Torres and Juan Fernandez, seeking passage for Sanchan Island and Goa. They sailed to Sanchan in 1551. Xavier had spent two rugged years in Japan during which he became captivated by the Japanese people. He was not disheartened by his relative lack of success there and continued to hold the conversion of the Japanese as his primary goal. Aware of the long centuries of Chinese influence in Japan, he concluded that if the Chinese could be brought into the Christian fold, the Japanese might follow suit. He left Almeida's ship at Sanchan and proceeded to Goa where he persuaded the governor and the provincial to establish a mission that would lead him to China. But he died at Sanchan on December 2, 1552, unsuccessful in his final efforts to enter China.

Almeida continued to trade between Siam, Malacca, Sanchan, and Japan. His bravery and his skill as a sailor were tested when the ship carrying the vice-provincial of the missions foundered in the straits of Johore off Singapore. Although the waters were the domain of Malayan pirates who detested the Portuguese, Almeida rescued all hands with no loss of life.

It was in 1555 that Almeida, still a young man of thirty years, decided to enter the Society of Jesus and apply his medical knowledge and his money toward the success of the Japanese mission. It was not uncommon for Portuguese laymen in the Far East to enter the society. In September of that year he wrote to a friend, Belchior Nunes, and requested that Nunes inform him in what manner he could best apply his money and his talent in the service of God. Almeida began his medical work in Japan at the hospital in Funai. This institution had been established by a Jesuit, Baltazar Gago, and named for a chapel in Lisbon where Trinitaire Miguel Contreros, founder of the Misericordia, had treated the sick poor.

The plight of the sick and the destitute touched Almeida deeply, and he gave freely of his medical skills and his money to ease their suffering. But he was especially concerned with the two groups that were shunned by their countrymen, the foundlings and the lepers. Infanticide and the desertion of children were rife, especially among the impoverished peasants, and Almeida gave 1,000 crusadoes for an orphanage for foundlings. He also undertook the care of the other pitiful group, the lepers, and opened a hospital for them in December, 1556; for this he received a measure of financial support from the lord of Bungo, Ōtomo Sōrin, which was in essence a bait for trade. At Ōtomo's urging, Almeida practiced medicine and surgery at a temple in Funai where he also taught about fifteen Japanese students, including two converts who had been baptized as Paul and Gregory.

In 1582 the visitor-general of the Jesuit missions in Japan and China, Alessandro Valignano, came to Japan and directed that henceforth any medical services would be restricted to the nobility and samurai; lepers and venereal patients would not be accepted under any circumstances. He was reverting to the well-established Jesuit policy that concentrated efforts on the rulers and leaders of a country. Also, Valignano probably felt that because of the remarkable success of the priests in converting the Japanese it would be advisable to concentrate activities on the missionary phases of the program rather than muddy the waters with a medical program. A third reason was that by offering medical care and shelter to foundlings and lepers the Jesuits might draw the hostility of the feudal lords, who had no concern for the health of the lower classes.

In 1565 the mikado at the behest of the bonzes decreed that all Jesuits must leave Japan, but because he was powerless the decree was not enforced. The great warrior-chieftain Oda Nobunaga befriended and supported the Jesuits because he detested the bonzes and was eager to maintain and expand trade with China, essentially all of which was carried in Portuguese hulls. After Nobunaga was assassinated in 1582, the military power fell to Toyotomi Hideyoshi, who for a time befriended the Jesuits. He respècted them but at the same time recognized that their preachings were contrary to the religion and therefore the welfare of his people. In 1587 he issued a decree that the Jesuits must leave Japan, but it was not enforced. The Jesuits retreated from the center of power in Kyoto to Nagasaki and there made every effort to avoid public religious display.

A second blow to the Jesuits fell about six years later, in 1593, when Spanish Franciscan friars from the Philippines entered Japan and established a missionary program. They had had their eye on Japan for some years and had looked on the Philippines simply as stepping stones for intensive programs in China and Japan. The Treaty of Tordesillas, proclaimed by Pope Alexander VI on June 7, 1494, established a line 370 leagues west of the Cape Verde Islands; the Portuguese were to have exclusive rights

Hideyoshi died in 1598. In contrast to his hatred of the bonzes, which encouraged his tolerance of the Christians, his successor, Tokugawa Ieyasu, was a practicing Buddhist. However, he was sufficiently involved with settling internal strife and with the development of trade so that for seventeen years he made no effort to enforce the previously published edicts of expulsion.

Meanwhile, the unique position of the Portuguese as the dominant Western nation in Japan was terminated by the arrival of the Hollanders.

The first Dutch reached Japan in April, 1600, drifting ashore on the *Liefde*, the sole surviving ship from a squadron of three which had traversed the Straits of Magellan and encountered violent storms. The pilot was an Englishman, Will Adams, who was summoned before Ieyasu and who by dint of his resourcefulness and information soon became Ieyasu's trusted adviser.

Ieyasu was eager to expand commerce and invited the Dutch to establish a trading post in Japan. In 1609 the Dutch flag was raised at Hirado Island, northwest of Nagasaki. Hirado Island had been an active trading port for the Portuguese; it was a good anchorage and had the advantage of being distant from Kyoto and Edo. Ten years later the headquarters of the Dutch Asian empire was established in Java on the ruins of the old fortress Djakarta. The post was named Batavia (now Djakarta) after the German tribe that first settled in The Netherlands, at the mouth of the Rhine.

In 1612 Ieyasu determined to rid his country of Christianity, and a new edict expelling all priests was promulgated. His primary reason was that he had decided to establish a completely feudal state, and the distractions occasioned by foreign flags would cause problems. A second reason was his concern for a possible revolt in which Japanese converts would join an invasion force from Spain or Portugal to seize the empire by force. A third reason was that Ieyasu realized he could maintain trade with Europe without the troublesome missionaries. After 1614 the edict was strictly enforced, and in 1622 there was a mass martyrdom at Nagasaki. Thirty Christians, including five European Dominicans, were burned alive and thirty-one beheaded. In 1624 all Spaniards were expelled.

Not all of the Christians withstood the agonies of persecution, and the first of seven Jesuit fathers to recant was a missionary-physician, Christavaõ Ferreira. Ferreira was born in Portugal in 1590 and came to Japan in 1611. In 1623, when he was the vice-provincial of the Jesuit mission, he apostasized after hanging head down over a pit of excreta for six hours. He then took a Japanese name, Sawano Chūan, and wrote several books on Western surgery: *Namban Geka Hidensho* [The secret book of southern barbarian surgery]; *Namban Chūan Geka Hidensho* [The secret book of Chūan's southern barbarian surgery]; and *Namban Geka-Shū* [A miscellany of the surgery of the southern barbarians]. Ferreira expounded the humoral theories of Galenic medicine and emphasized the importance of plasters and ointments in external infections. One of the earliest Western astronomy texts to appear in Japan was *Kenkon Bensetsu* [Heaven and earth speech theory], which was a translation by Chūan of a Portuguese book on astronomy.

During the first quarter of the seventeenth century the study of plants for medicinal purposes (*honzō-gaku*) was expanded. As early as the eighth century a Chinese text from the T'ang dynasty, *Hsin-hsiu pên-ts'ao* (also *Shinshūhonzō*) [Newly reorganized pharmacopoeia], was brought to Japan. In 1613 an important book on botany and natural history, *Pên-ts'ao-kang-mu* (also *Honzō-kōmoku*), written in China in 1596 by Li Shih-ch'en, reached Japan. Its fifty-two volumes included descriptions of more than one thousand plants, animals, and minerals; the major emphasis was on plants. In the same year Ieyasu, who was interested in the cultivation of medicinal plants in his garden at Edo castle, ordered Hayashi Razan, a member of the famed Hayashi family of scholars, to write a series of books on medicinal plants. These were entitled *Tashikihen*, *Honzō Kōmoku Kyōchū*, and *Honzō Joreichū* and were derived from the *Pên-ts'ao-kang-mu*.

From 1633 to 1636 a series of edicts calling for *sakoku* ("closed country") was issued. The first of these was addressed to the two governors of Nagasaki, and its major provisions were that no vessels could sail for a foreign port without a license, no Japanese could leave the country without a permit, and any Japanese returning from abroad would be executed.

In 1634 the shogun Tokugawa Iemitsu decided to isolate the only remaining Iberians, a handful of Portuguese traders, in one place at Nagasaki and ordered the twenty-five leading merchants in the city to fill in the rocky shore in front of the Portuguese factory at Edo-machi. The merchants were further directed to erect warehouses and living quarters—at their own expense. The Portuguese traders were moved to the man-made island of Deshima in 1636, but two years later they too were banished to Macao.

Iemitsu was now firm in his intention to close the country, yet "the Tokugawa were wise enough not to cut off all contact with other nations. They preserved Nagasaki as a window looking out on the rest of the world" (Reischauer, 1946, p. 91). While her neighbor and cultural mother, China, stood aloof from all contacts, the island-nation of Japan recognized the advantage of maintaining contact with the West. Here we should note that the first contacts between China and the West and between Japan and the West were quite different. In China the Portuguese did not hesitate to burn, pillage, sack, and bombard. In Japan, on the other hand, the dominant personality in the early contacts was St. Francis Xavier; the Portuguese did not resort to force in Japan. In China the harquebus (a portable firearm) symbolized the first contacts—in Japan the symbol was the crucifix.

Having made the decision to maintain contact with the West, the Japanese had no choice but the Dutch with whom to maintain it. A British trading post on Hirado Island was short-lived and closed in 1623 because of mismanagement and keen competition from the Dutch. In contrast to the banished Portuguese and Spaniards, the Hollanders had concentrated on trade and had sedulously avoided any sign of missionary activity. Merchants from the *godaisho-kaisho* ("five trading places")—Sakai, Osaka, Kyoto, Edo, and Nagasaki—urged the shogunate to move the Dutch to Nagasaki so that they would be more accessible to trade.

The Hollanders were moved from Hirado Island to Deshima on June 18, 1641, and this little island became "the window looking out on the rest of the world."

19

弐

CHAPTER

II

The Early Years at Deshima:
Willem Ten Rhijne and Engelbert Kaempfer

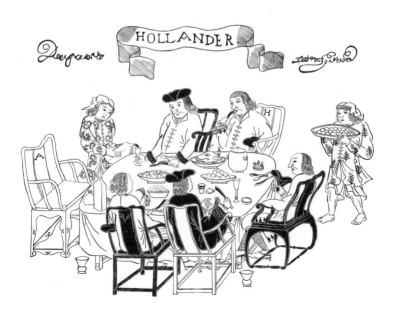

DESHIMA WAS A small fan-shaped island 197 feet wide; it measured 557 feet along its northern shore and 706 feet along the southern shore, with a total area of thirty-two acres. In 1641 the island was crowded with several hundred vigilant Japanese attending a handful of Dutchmen. It was surrounded by a tall wooden fence, and the main entrance, at the midpoint of the northern shore, was connected to the mainland by a short stone bridge. There was a guardhouse at the main entrance, and a floodgate on the west side was usually barred except when the ships came from Batavia to trade. Thirteen boundary piles in the surrounding waters warned all ships to keep their distance. At night the sleep of the Hollanders was disturbed by hourly Japanese patrols that made their presence known by beating loudly on drums. Even the gutters were serpentine to prevent secret exchanges with the outside.

Fortunately for posterity, the Hollanders and their island prison were favorite subjects of Japanese artists. The prints of Deshima show two narrow streets lined by forty-four buildings, including up to thirty warehouses with living quarters on the second floor. There were about a dozen residences, including homes for the *opperhoofd*, the doctor and other Hollanders, and the Japanese town chief. Other buildings housed offices, shops, and community facilities. By the main gate there was a large botanical garden. A second-floor entertainment pavilion is always shown crowded with Hollanders and geisha.

The prints depict vividly the life of the average Hollander at Deshima. Content to waste his days and nights, he lolls in a large chair, smoking a long pipe and looking very bored. A table loaded with food is before him, a decanter and glasses at one arm and a fawning geisha at the other. The ever-watchful Nagasaki interpreters are kneeling on the far side of the room, and scurrying Javanese foot servants are in the background.

The Japanese artists always adorned the Hollanders with red hair or a red periwig and dubbed them *kōmō* ("red hairs"); this name was intended to suggest diabolical beings more than hair color. The Hollanders were for many years considered supernatural creatures by the Japanese, like goblins or demons, with no heels, and it was rumored that when they urinated, they raised a leg like a dog. The large, round eyes of the Hollanders impressed the Japanese children, who shouted *Oranda-ō-me* ("Dutch-big-eyes") when the strangers appeared on the streets of Nagasaki.

The handful of Hollanders at Deshima included the *opperhoofd* and his deputy, a doctor, a few clerks, and several artisans. They were guarded, watched, and assisted by more than two hundred Japanese, including interpreters, accountants, landlords, cooks, and guards. The Japanese limited the tour of duty for the *opperhoofd* to one year so that he would not be able to acquire detailed information about the country. However, the *opperhoofd* could return after an absence of one year, and several of them, such as Camphuijs and Titsingh, did so in order to study the culture of Japan. Others returned for more practical reasons— the *opperhoofd* also served as captain of a highly lucrative smuggling operation.

Signboards on the narrow streets of Deshima were posted with the harsh regulations that governed the Dutch:

STRICT IMPERIAL COMMANDS:

1. Our Imperial Predecessors have order'd concerning you Dutchmen, that you shall have leave to come to Nagasaki, on account of the Japanese trade, every year . . . you shall have no communication with the Portuguese. If you should have any, and we should come to know of it from foreign countries, you shall be prohibited the navigation to Japan. You shall import no Portuguese commodities. . . .

2. . . . You shall notify to us by your ships, whatever comes to your knowledge, of any endeavors or attempts of the Portuguese against us; . . . if the Portuguese should conquer any new places or countries, or convert them to the Christian Sect. Whatever comes to your knowledge in all countries you trade to, we expect that you should notify the same to our Governor at Nagasaki.

3. You shall take no Chinese junks bound for Japan.

4. In all countries you frequent with your ships, if there be any Portuguese there, you shall have no communication with them.

Regulations concerning the street Deshima:

Whores only, but no other Women, shall be suffer'd to go in.

23

Only the Ecclesiasticks of the mountain *Kōja* shall be admitted. All other priests and all *Jammabos* shall stand excluded.*

All beggars, and all persons that live upon charity shall be denied Entrance.

No body shall presume, with any ship or boat, to come within the Pallisadoes of Deshima.

No Hollander shall be permitted to come out, but for weighty reasons" [Kaempfer, 1727, 1: 383–84].

As the imperial commands indicate, the Japanese retained an abiding fear of the Portuguese and the possible restoration of Christian missions. When the Dutch ships approached the road-stead at Nagasaki, in addition to transferring guns and ammunition to Deshima, the captain sequestered all Bibles, prayer books, and other evidences of Christianity until the ships departed for Batavia. As an example of the overwhelming anxieties of the Japanese, when a drunken Dutch sailor fell overboard in Naga-saki Bay, the attendant commotion immediately aroused Japa-nese suspicions that he was a Portuguese Jesuit fleeing to the countryside to preach the forbidden faith. The officers of the guard were so overwhelmed by the magnitude of their possible dereliction of duty that they began to strip aside their robes in preparation for ripping up their bellies. They were spared a ritualistic *seppuku* only after the sailor was hauled aboard and identified as a Hollander.

Each New Year every citizen of Nagasaki was required to publicly demonstrate his anti-Christian sentiments by performing *fumiye*—trampling on a metal plate that bore an image of the Virgin Mary and the cross. For infants too young to walk, mothers complied with the edict by rubbing the tiny feet on the metal plate.

To further seal the country against the infiltration of Christi-anity, the shogun Tokugawa Iemitsu in 1630 banned thirty-two

* *Kōja* (also *Gyōja*) priests were Buddhists from a mountain near Kyoto who were not under the strict restrictions on travel which applied to the other orders—they were allowed to travel freely. *Jammabos* (also *Yamabushi*), members of another Buddhist sect, aggressively combative and independent, were openly defiant of the government.

scientific and religious books written or translated into Chinese by Jesuits and converts in China, principally the writings of the distinguished Jesuit scholar Father Matthew Ricci. The translations included Euclid's *Elements* and Cicero's *On Friendship*, as well as treatises on astronomy and geography. The Japanese were especially apprehensive over a series of provocative tracts that Father Ricci had written on Christianity; they were imaginary dialogues in Chinese between a European Roman Catholic priest and a Chinese scholar.

Father Ricci was an Italian Jesuit who came to the coast of China in 1582 after four years in Goa and Cochin. His missionary program was based on the belief that the Chinese door to Christianity would be most readily opened by teaching European sciences—especially mathematics, physics, and geography—to the leaders and gentry. He learned to speak and read Chinese and he translated Western mathematics texts to enhance the effectiveness of this teaching. To further ingratiate himself with the Chinese he donned the robes of a mandarin. Father Ricci, a skilled craftsman, made sundials and globes and corrected the maps and astronomical charts of the court at Peking.

By banning the books of the Jesuits, the Japanese essentially cut themselves off from ready access to the achievements of Western science and technology, since Chinese was their only foreign tongue. An occasional book in Dutch was brought into the country, but for more than one hundred years only the interpreters at Nagasaki had any facility in Dutch and their ability was decidedly limited.

The bans on books should have closed all access to Western science and medicine, but no ban could diminish the abiding curiosity of Japanese scholars for new ideas and innovations. They turned to Nagasaki and the Dutch as the one source of information on the wider world.

The life of the doctor at Deshima was such as to satisfy a variety of tastes. For the physician who was a rover there was the attraction of a long sea voyage from Amsterdam with ports of call at Cape Colony (now the Cape of Good Hope), Malabar, the East Indies, and Siam before reaching Japan. For the scholar there was the opportunity to study a fascinating, unique, and

25

admirable culture and, in turn, to transmit to eager Japanese students his own fund of knowledge. For the rake there was the opportunity to keep a Japanese prostitute and to visit the nearby famed Maruyama geisha quarter, where the beauty of the girls was surpassed only by the geisha in the Gion quarter of Kyoto.* Since the Hollanders were not permitted to bring their wives to Japan, there was no fear of domestic reprisal for illicit romances, and many Dutchmen enjoyed the pleasures of a solicitous and obedient Japanese concubine.

The monotony of the doctor's life could be broken by occasional passes to botanize in the environs of Nagasaki, but he was always escorted by a number of Japanese guards for whom he was obliged to purchase food and drink at a considerable expense.

Deshima was hardly attractive to the physician interested in the care of the sick. There simply were not enough patients to keep him active in medicine. When he was asked to consult on a Japanese patient it was usually through an interpreter serving as middleman, and the doctor was not permitted to see or examine the patient.

Given the variety of opportunities and problems at Deshima, it was only natural that the doctors ranged from barber-surgeons, whom Thunberg described as little better than horse doctors, to a few—Ten Rhijne, Kaempfer, Thunberg, and Siebold—who were scholars and scientists. It was these four men who studied the Japanese culture, collected materials representing the botany, natural history, and the arts of Japan for exhibit and study in Europe, and through their writings and collections became the leading Western scholars on Japan during the centuries of closure to the West.

Each August, Japanese sentinels on the mountainous island that the Dutch called Papenberg would light the signal fires to show that a foreign vessel was entering Nagasaki harbor.†

* The attractions of Maruyama continue today, and the finest of the old geisha houses (Kagetsu) is a favorite place of entertainment for the wealthier men of Nagasaki. The beautiful wooden posts at Kagetsu show deep gashes made by the samurai when demonstrating their prowess with the long sword to impress the geisha.

† The promontory was said to have acquired the name Papenberg because from it many Portuguese Catholics were thrown to their deaths.

Shortly an East Indiaman flying the beautiful Dutch tricolor appeared with guns booming a salute, but her glory was short-lived, for almost immediately, by Japanese regulation, her rudder was shipped, not only to ensure navigational safety, but also to prevent any hostile maneuvers. Under human tow she was moved to the anchorage near Deshima. If there was concern about the identification of a vessel, the first signal fire was followed by a series stretching to Edo so that within twenty-four hours the shogun was informed of trouble at Nagasaki.

Deshima was at first the most lucrative trading post in the far-flung Dutch empire because of the rich Japanese deposits of silver, gold, and copper. The profits from this trade were usually at least 50 per cent and in 1670 they mounted as high as 70 per cent. But after 1685, because of dwindling reserves of the metals and public apprehension over financial policies, the export of silver was prohibited and only two Dutch ships were permitted to enter Nagasaki each year. Gold, copper, rice, lacquer ware, pottery, camphor, and sake were the major export items; but in time the export of gold and copper was also probihited.

Medicines were always a major import item, and at the beginning of the eighteenth century a leading official of the shogun's court stated that they were the only essential item: "With the exception of medicines, we can dispense with everything that is brought us from abroad. . . . other foreign commodities are of no real benefit to us" (Titsingh, 1822, pp. 28–29).

"Unicorn" horns were a popular medicine imported by the Dutch and were purported to be life-prolonging, but their therapeutic value had not been established. The horns were in fact those of East African elephants or the single tusk of the narwhal (*Monodon monoceros*) of the arctic seas: "The Japanese have an extraordinary opinion of its medical virtues and powers to prolong the life, fortify the animal spirits, assist the memory and cure all complaints" (Thunberg, 1795, 3:49).

The Hollanders were able to supply the Japanese with other compounds believed to have medicinal value. These were collected from the many ports where their vessels traded—from Amsterdam to Africa, the Middle East, India, the Spice Islands, Siam, and Formosa—and included bezoars, gall stones of oxen and wild boars, a sweet-scented balm from Arabia called *mommie*, saffron, as well as a number of compounds used in Batavia, such as "Dutch cough cure."

The crowning event of the year for the Dutch was the annual *hofreis* to Edo to present to the shogun the *fūsetsusho* ("annual report") on the state of all countries where the Hollanders traded and the activities of the Portuguese. By Japanese tradition they were also required to present costly gifts. The *hofreis* followed the edict that all *daimyō* report to the shogun at Edo each year on the state of their fiefs. It was a great financial burden to the Hollanders, for the cost of maintaining the large Japanese retinue and the numerous gifts usually exceeded sixty thousand guldens. After 1790 the *hofreis* was made quadrennial because Dutch trade had declined, and only the captain, doctor, and chief clerk made the journey.

The *hofreis* was a splendid opportunity for the Hollanders to see Japan: her verdant mountains and gentle coastlines; her terraced farms with paddies occupying every tillable foot of land; her crowded cities; her magnificent temples and shrines; and her diligent, courteous, and inquisitive people. The accounts of the *hofreis* conjure up a fascinating picture of a long and colorful procession of a few Dutchmen, guarded by more than two hundred Japanese, winding its way by land and by sea from Nagasaki to Edo. Before leaving Nagasaki the Japanese took a blood oath to report to the governor any infringement of the laws and instructions by the Dutch. These laws and instructions required that the Dutch should be incommunicado throughout the sojourn. Nevertheless, several of the doctors recorded detailed information on Japan, including maps of the countryside and sketches of public buildings, and assembled extensive collections of botanical and zoological specimens, all with the assistance of the Japanese.

The Interpreters

The first Japanese to be taught Western surgery and medicine at Deshima were the *Orandatsūji* ("Dutch interpreters"). In exchange they were quite willing to inform the Hollanders about the culture, medicine, and geography of Japan. The interpreters had picked up a smattering of medicine from the Portuguese, but with the advent of the Hollanders they turned to the study of medicine more seriously. In addition to their role as interpreters, they served as traders and spies. By government order, after 1671 the Dutch gave the interpreters formal instruction at Deshima in reading and writing Dutch. In time the interpreters taught medicine and Dutch to other Japanese who were sent to Nagasaki by their *daimyō*.

For close to half a century the relations between the Hollanders and the interpreters were strained. The latter held a lingering affection for the Portuguese, and the language of the Lusitanians continued to be the *lingua franca* until the turn of the century. The Hollanders naturally resented not only their dependence on the interpreters for communication but also the fact that the interpreters spied on them. Even fifty years after the Dutch first came to Deshima, Kaempfer found the interpreters "most prejudicial to our honour, liberty and welfare" (1727, 1:345).

The leading families of interpreters were the Nishi, Motoki, Narabayashi, and Yoshio, all of whom established medical dynasties. Perhaps the most famous was the Narabayashi family, beginning with Narabayashi Chinzan (also known as Shingohei) (1643–1711). He studied under Willem Hoffman, who was the doctor at Deshima from 1671 to 1675, and then left his post as interpreter to become a full-time practitioner and teacher of Western medicine. In 1706 Narabayashi published *Kōi geka sōden* (also *Kōmō geka sōden*) [Dutch surgery handed down], a six-volume work written in Chinese. Of special interest is the third volume, *Kinsō tetsuboku zu*, which explains surgical procedures and bandaging and includes a number of plates showing European surgical instruments. The illustrations so closely resemble those of Ambroise Paré's *De chirurgie* that it has been suggested that Narabayashi copied from Paré. However, the book was probably a combination of Paré and information that Narabayashi acquired at Deshima. In his fourth introductory remark Narabayashi explains that the therapeutic methods of Dutch internal medicine were abbreviated in his translation since they were of no significance to the Japanese—Western surgery was the principal interest. Another book, *Kinsō Tetsuboku Ryōji*, derived from Paré, was published in 1713 by Gentetsu Nishi.

The first Western doctor whose name appears in the annals as a teacher was Caspar Schamberger, a barber-surgeon of German origin. Just eight years after Japan was closed to the West he was instructing four Japanese youths in the treatment of wounds. Schamberger had come to Nagasaki in 1650 with a singularly important mission occasioned by the shogun's refusal to accept the annual gifts from the Dutch because they had signed a treaty with the hated Portuguese. As an indication of the importance that the Dutch attached to the Nagasaki trade, an embassy was sent out from Amsterdam led by a distinguished doctor of law, Peter Blockhovius. Unfortunately he was chosen for his years as well as his diplomatic abilities and he expired on the long voyage. However, his successor, Frisius, was able to persuade the *bakufu* that the Portuguese contact was of no consequence, and normal relations were restored.

Schamberger's system was based on the use of external ointments, poultices, and plasters. These are described in an anonymous manual, *Kōmō-geka* [Surgery of the red hairs]. The emphasis on external applications was in contrast to the traditional reliance on internal medications in *Kampō*.

When Schamberger accompanied the *opperhoofd* on the *hofreis*, he received so much attention from the Japanese physicians that from then on the doctor was always a member of the Dutch delegation on the annual visit to the shogun's capital.

The Japanese wrote several treatises on Schamberger's surgical methods. Inomata Dembei, one of the interpeters who studied with him, published *Kaspar-ryū-i-sho* [Medical book of the Caspar school] and *Oranda-geka-sho* [Dutch book of surgery]. In 1661 Kawaguchi Ryōan published *Caspar dempō*.

Even the officials of the shogunate at Edo took steps to obtain information on Western medicine and botany. In 1650 the *bakufu* ordered the Dutch mission to bring to Edo a book on Western anatomy and four years later they directed a Nagasaki physician, Mukai Genshō (1609–77), to compile information on the surgical methods of the Dutch. Mukai had studied under *opperchirurgien* Hans Jonson and wrote *Kōmō-ryū-geka-hōmō* [Secret outlines of red-haired school surgery]. Also in 1654 one of the officials of the shogunate, Inoue Chikugo-no-kami, undertook the translation into Portuguese of several Dutch anatomical texts. Five years later, at the request of the *rōjū* ("council of elders"), the *opperhoofd*, Zacharias Wagenaer, included in the annual gifts a Western botany text, *Herbarius oft Cruijdt-Boeck* (1618), by the great botanist Rembertus Dodonaeus, a professor at Leiden.

In 1663 the *opperhoofd*, Hendrick Indijck, presented an encyclopedic book on animals, *Beschrijveng van de Natuur der Viervoetige Dieren, Vissen en Bloedloze Waterdieren Vogelen, Kronkeldieren Slangen en Draken*, by Jan Johnston, to the court.

Daniel Busch, a surgeon at Deshima from 1662 to 1666, was probably the first Deshima doctor whom Nagasaki officials authorized to give medical care to the people of their city. That he was an active teacher as well is attested to by the appearance of his name on the first certificate of proficiency in medicine. It was awarded to Arashiyama Hōan in 1665 and is retained in the museum at Hirado Island:

> We, the undersigned, bear witness and attest as the truth that the Japanese named *Chōan*, servant of the lord of Hirado, has studied for a considerable time under the Dutch surgeons and is well instructed (so far as we can tell) in the art of Surgery. He is therefore well acquainted with the potency of Dutch medicines, of which he has given us sufficient practical proofs, and we hereby declare him to be an accomplished practitioner.—JAPAN, in the agency of Nagasaki, this 21st January, 1665. (signed) Jacob Gruijs. 1665. Nicolaes de Roy, D. Busch, surgeon, on the island of Deshima [Boxer, 1950, p. 46].

In 1683 the same Arashiyama Hōan, who was now a physician at Hirado Island, published *Shinkokujihō Ruishū* [Compilation of various foreign methods of treatment], which was used as a text for a number of years by Japanese who came to Deshima to study Western medicine and surgery. Two years later Nakamura Sōyō, who had come from Kyoto to study at Deshima, published *Geka-Ryōji-Shū*, another report on Western surgery as practiced at Deshima.

Willem Ten Rhijne

The first Deshima doctor to describe the medicine and culture of Japan to the West was a Hollander, Willem Ten Rhijne. There

31

had been brief notes on the unique practices of *Kampō* in the letters of the Jesuits, such as those of Father Luis Frois (see Chapter I), but Ten Rhijne was the first physician to publish in Europe a detailed description of the indications for and practices of acupuncture and moxibustion. He was as well the first physician with a full university education in medicine to come to Deshima, and his studies and publications indicate that he was dedicated to scholarship.

Ten Rhijne was born in 1647 at the trading center Deventer, to Anna Petrus, an unmarried mother. As a resident of one of the northern Dutch provinces where Protestants were dominant, Ten Rhijne had every opportunity for a good education. After the separation from Spain, strong primary schools attached to Calvinist churches and Latin upper schools were established in the north. Ten Rhijne studied in Deventer at the Illustre School, whose greatest student had been the leading humanist of the Renaissance, Erasmus. After upper school at Franeker in Friesland, Ten Rhijne enrolled as a student in the medical faculty at the University of Leiden. The university had risen to eminence rapidly by pioneering in the development of an educational program in engineering, a botanical garden, an astronomical observatory, and the famed Elsevier University Press, all of which were based on strong traditional faculties of law and medicine.

The medical faculty in Ten Rhijne's student days was led by Franz de la Böe (1614–72), better known by his Latin name, Franciscus Sylvius. As a professor of medicine, Sylvius was a pioneer of the school of iatrochemistry, which moved medicine from Galenic dogma to a recognition that health and disease are based on the chemistry of the body. Sylvius proposed that fermentation was the primary chemical process of the body. Perhaps his chemical interests in fermentation led him to another important contribution—the development of gin, which he hoped would prevent or cure the fevers that were so prevalent in the Dutch fleets. Sylvius was a leader in the development of clinical bedside teaching north of the Alps and, since the United Provinces practiced fewer religious discriminations than other countries in Europe, students from across the continent flocked to Leiden.

After two years as a student at Leiden, Ten Rhijne presented his dissertation, "De Dolore Intestinorum e Flatu," and was awarded the doctorate in medicine. He then exhibited the devotion to writing which characterized his life; in 1669 he published two treatises at Leiden, *Dissertatio de Arthritide* and *Meditationes in Magni Hippocratis de veteri medicina.* In the former he discussed joint pains and their possible causes and in the latter he wrote of the then current concepts of bodily functions: pneumazologia, phytologia, and chymologia.

In June, 1673, Ten Rhijne sailed from Holland on the *Ternate,* and four months later his ship dropped anchor at Table Bay to provision at the Dutch colony that had been established twenty years earlier. The seventeen directors of the Dutch East India Company, the Heeren 17, had been concerned about the high incidence of fevers and malnutrition in the fleet and had established Cape Colony with the hope that fresh food and fresh air would improve the health of the sailors.

Ten Rhijne's ability as a perceptive observer is clearly demonstrated by the volume and variety of information which he gathered on the fascinating Hottentots during the little more than three weeks that he spent at the Cape in 1686. As a good Calvinist he was shocked by what he described as their evil way of life, their lust and licentiousness. The relations of the Hottentot women with the Hollanders were varied: one Hottentot woman had hanged herself because a Dutchman had debauched her; another was happily married to a Dutch surgeon; a third, being fluent in both Portuguese and Dutch, served the Dutch as an interpreter.

The women appeared "for the most part naked, having only a piece of leather, like an apron hanging from their breasts." "Out of their Privities you see two Labels hanging down like part of a Man's Yard of these they are very proud . . . and show them to the stranger" (Churchill, 1774, pp. 835–36).* When a woman was delivered of twins, the second was always killed. Marriage was perfunctory; the women cut off as many joints from their fingers as they had husbands, beginning with the first joint of the little finger. Soon after birth one of the testicles was cut out of all

* These were actually the *labia minora,* which had been stretched from infancy.

male children in the belief that this would enable them to run more swiftly. Copulation was usually performed from behind.

The medicine of the Hottentots relied almost exclusively on suction and on unctions made with beef or mutton suet. The sources and natures of their medicines were held secret; for example, abdominal colic was cured with a root which they refused to identify. The governor of the colony had a stone from a human testicle mounted as a jewel on a ring but in a diplomatic move presented it to a native chief who wished to wear it as an antidote.

The peculiar clicking speech of the Hottentots reminded Ten Rhijne of the myths about a Pythagorean age when the birds conversed.*

Ten Rhijne did not limit his observations to the Hottentots; *Schediasma de Promontorio Bonaespei* opens with a discussion of the southeast winds at Table Bay, which always posed navigational problems and at times made the anchorage unsafe. He gathered an extensive collection of botanical specimens which he subsequently catalogued and published. His treatise on the Hottentots "probably helped more than any other of his works to make his name known in foreign countries" (translated from Dorssen, p. 6).

From the Cape the *Ternate* sailed across the roaring forties to Batavia—as usual, a miserable voyage of two months. On arrival Ten Rhijne was assigned to teach anatomy to the surgeons at Java; six months later, on June 20, 1674, he set sail for Japan with the new *opperhoofd*, Martinus Caesar.

The circumstances under which Ten Rhijne went to Japan are unclear. Drakestein states, "On the command of the Emperor of Japan he was sent by the Dutch East India Company because of his knowledge won abroad" (translated from van Reede tot Drakestein, p. 66), while the 1885 lexicon of Gurlt and Hirsch reports, "he was called to offer medical aid to the sick Emperor, and is said to have cured the latter" (translated from Gurlt *et al.*, 1932, p. 787). We know that Ten Rhijne was the first physician at Deshima to hold a university degree, and when he made the *hofreis* he undoubtedly was consulted by physicians from the

* The language of the Hottentots is monosyllabic and tonal and about 75 per cent of the words begin with a click.

mikado's court at Kyoto and the shogun's court at Edo. But it is doubtful that there was a request specifically for Ten Rhijne, because he had gained little, if any, recognition.

Unfortunately, we do not have a detailed account of Ten Rhijne's studies in Japan, but it is clear from the number and variety of his subsequent publications that he was an active and perceptive student of the medicine and botany of the empire, despite severe restrictions on his activities.

Ten Rhijne was the author of the first detailed descriptions of the practices of Chinese and Japanese medicine to appear in the West. These were published in 1683, seven years after he left Japan, in an unusual book, *Dissertatio de Arthritide*. It opens with a poetic dialogue written by a gouty, grateful patient of Ten Rhijne's, Reverend Herman Busschof, a pastor at Batavia. The dialogue is between Busschof and a person named Podagra. *Podagra* ("foot-catching") was the name first applied to gout by the Greeks because of its frequent involvement of the big toe. It was also the name of a lesser goddess born of the seduction of Aphrodite by Dionysius. From this latter relationship of Podagra sprang in part the emphasis on sex and gout which Hippocrates laid down: A young man does not take the gout unless he indulges in coitus; eunuchs do not take the gout nor become bald; woman does not take the gout unless her menses be stopped. In the dialogue the pastor discusses the manifestations of gout and mentions the use of acupuncture and moxibustion.

Acupuncture is described by Ten Rhijne as especially useful in treating "illnesses of the belly and stomach as well as illness of the head." The needles, which were almost always of gold—rarely of silver, and never of any other metal—were introduced by a twisting motion or by tapping them gently with a hammer. Ten Rhijne noted that the people of Hindustan and Arakan used a rather similar needle to remove harmful vapors from the body; thus, he added, the Brahmins, the Chinese, and the Japanese are the fellow workers of Hippocrates, *"de Flatibus Passim."*

For moxibustion, the leaves of *Artemisia vulgaris* were stripped from their fibers and rolled into small balls the size of a pea or into cylinders to be sliced before application. Ten Rhijne reported that the Chinese usually wrapped the moxa in cloth, then

35

moistened the site of the application, applied the moxa, ignited it, and covered it with a wooden cup. The treatment was painless and it was necessary to cover the eschar with a plantago leaf for only twenty-four hours. And, as is true today, the Japanese used moxa not only for the gout but for many other diseases as well. There are two additional essays in *Dissertatio de Arthritide*: one describes the characteristics of arthritis and the other serves as a postscript to the poetic dialogue. The book includes a number of plates of both Japanese and Chinese origin, several of which show on exotic human forms the sites for the application of the moxa or the insertion of the acupuncture needles.

Willem Ten Rhijne was responsible for the first descriptions and specimens of the tea plant to come to the West. Just a few months after his arrival at Nagasaki he sent an essay on the tea plant, a branch of a camphor tree, and a batch of twigs, leaves, and flowers representative of the flora of Japan to an old friend, Jacobus Breynius, a Danzig botanist. The essay, with an excellent sketch of the tea plant, was added to a list of plants at Cape Colony compiled by Ten Rhijne and was published in a collection by Breynius in 1678. Kaempfer later described this essay on the tea plant as "prolix and accurate" (1727, vol. 2, app. 1, p. 1). He noted that Ten Rhijne led a more restricted life at Deshima than his successors and did not have the same opportunities to study Japan.

Ten Rhijne made the *hofreis* to Edo on two occasions, and on the second the *opperhoofd* was Johannes Camphuijs, who later became the governor general at Batavia.

Ten Rhijne sailed from Nagasaki on October 27, 1676, and reached Batavia on December 13 of that year. In Java, where he spent the rest of his life, he had a varied and productive career. His principal work was with leprosy, which was still a major scourge throughout the Far East. He was director of the leprosarium in Batavia and later a member of a commission appointed by the Dutch East India Company to make recommendations on the control of leprosy. The culmination of Ten Rhijne's studies on leprosy was the publication of *Verhandelinge Van de Asiatise Melaatsheid* in 1687. It has been described as the best work on the subject before 1830 (Broes van Dort). Although leprosy, for still

36

unknown reasons, had begun to disappear in Europe, the book was of special interest there because Ten Rhijne described in detail the many bizarre theories on the etiology of the disease and the unique methods of treatment popular in a number of Asian countries. One of the latter was moxibustion.

Unfortunately for Ten Rhijne, he crossed swords with an interesting and difficult man, Andreas Cleyer, who had served as *opperhoofd* at Deshima. A German from Kassel in Hesse-Nassau Province, Cleyer had taken an abbreviated program in medicine as a secondary doctor and was designated as licentiate or *doctorandus*. He first appeared at Batavia on July 8, 1664, as a professional soldier in The Netherlands East Indies Army. The variety of Cleyer's appointments included director of the *lycée*, chief pharmacist, and chief chemist in the government. He became head of the government medical section in 1676 and was influential in the expansion of the pharmaceutical program.

In 1682 Cleyer went to Deshima as *opperhoofd* for a year and returned for a second tour in 1685. But his success in smuggling made him too self-confident and his illegal activities became so apparent that he was finally expelled by the Japanese.

Smuggling was not Cleyer's only transgression. In 1682 he published *Specimen Medicinae Sinicae*, in which he plagiarized one of the earliest descriptions of Chinese medicine and botany, that by a Polish Jesuit, Michael Boym (1612–59). Boym, who reached China in 1649, had more than a passing knowledge of medicine because his father had served as physician to the king of Poland. After his death, Boym's manuscripts had been sent to Batavia by his colleague Father Couplet, and Cleyer seized them for his own use. They included discussions of the pulse theory of Chinese medicine, Chinese anatomy, and the diagnostic value of the tongue. Fortunately, an authentic edition bearing the name of Father Boym as author, but with another title, appeared in 1686.

The first *Flora Japonica* was published by Cleyer in Berlin and was illustrated with the drawings of Japanese plants which he had collected during his two tours as *opperhoofd*.

Ten Rhijne incurred Cleyer's wrath by making purportedly critical comments about a treatise that he had written on leprosy. Cleyer then seized every opportunity to abuse Ten Rhijne publicly, accusing him of dishonesty and unreliability. However, Cleyer's erratic traits were well-recognized; Ten Rhijne weathered the storm and died peacefully at Batavia on June 1, 1700.

Ten Rhijne was the only Dutch physician who made significant contributions to Western knowledge of Japan during the two centuries that the Hollanders held Deshima. The pioneering spirit of the Dutch was short-lived, and by the end of the seventeenth century they had forsaken exploration and adventure for the financial satisfaction of trade and comforts in Amsterdam and Haarlem; as the affluence of the citizens of Holland mounted, the financial attractions for a physician to remain in The Netherlands as a practitioner and teacher became even greater.

Half of the sailors in the hulls of the Dutch East India Company were foreign nationals led by Germans fleeing the ravages of the Thirty Years' War and, in smaller numbers, Swedes. So it was that in 1690, just fourteen years after Ten Rhijne left Nagasaki, a remarkable young German physician, scholar, and explorer, Engelbert Kaempfer, arrived in Deshima, thereby culminating eight years of travel and study in Sweden, Russia, Persia, Malabar, and Siam.

Engelbert Kaempfer

When Engelbert Kaempfer came to Nagasaki in 1690 at the age of thirty-nine, he was entering the climax of a fascinating career of scholarly inquiry, exploration, and adventure. His previous studies and experiences had prepared him in a unique manner for the task of gathering the remarkable body of information which he subsequently set down in his monumental legacy, *The History of Japan*. It is the most thorough and widely quoted source of information on the history and culture of Japan during the closed centuries of the Tokugawa shogunate.

Yet Kaempfer did not enjoy the satisfaction of seeing his book in print. The manuscript was written in German while he was practicing in Westphalia, but it was not published until after his death; it was translated into English and printed in London under the auspices of the president of the Royal Society and the Royal College of Physicians Sir Hans Sloane. Had it not been for the interest of Sir Hans it is possible that *The History of Japan* would never have been published. The German version, which appeared fifty years after the original English edition, is a translation of the English translation.

Despite the prison-like life at Deshima (broken by two opportunities to make the *hofreis* to Edo), Kaempfer collected a remarkable amount of information on Japan. The wide range of subjects that he studied included the mythological and actual history of the empire and the geography, climate, agriculture, natural history, mineral wealth, religions, government, and medicine of the country. His collections included maps, charts, numerous illustrations of the flora and fauna, as well as specimens from botany and natural history. They indicate that here was a man with a truly remarkable variety of talents—a scholar, a collector, an artist, a linguist, a physician, a scientist, and an explorer. He was the epitome of the Renaissance man.

At the time of Kaempfer's arrival Japan was in the Genroku era, 1688–1704, an era characterized by a wave of prosperity and bustling activity. The *bakufu* and the great lords had turned their attention from war to improving the economy, and major increases in agricultural productivity had resulted from extensive irrigation, intensive cultivation, and sound organization. The cities and towns were busy with manufacturing and trade. A spirit of intellectual inquiry was growing. There was a deep interest in Chinese art and culture and a lively creativity in poetry and painting. The emphasis in medicine continued to be on the study of the Chinese medical classics, the list being headed by *Shang Han Lun*, an ancient text written during the Han dynasty.

The prosperity and activity in Japan were in striking contrast to the wretched state of Kaempfer's homeland. Germany was a shambles from the devastating Thirty Years' War. Industry and commerce had been ruined; agriculture was at a standstill; the peasants were completely dependent upon the will of the great lords. Intellectual life and education had suffered severely, for the tragic conditions made material interests and the struggle for daily bread predominant.

Kaempfer was born on September 16, 1651, the third son of Johannes Kaempfer, who was the pastor of Nikolai Lutheran Church in the lovely little Hanseatic agricultural village of Lemgo, duchy of Lippe, Westphalia. At one time Lemgo had been the capital of the duchy, but because of the strong Lutheran sentiments in Lemgo, the Catholic prince moved to Detmold, just ten kilometers away. Nevertheless, Lemgo prospered as a member of the Hanse and shipped her farm products to Bremen, Flanders, and the Baltic Provinces. Her wealthy merchants lived in richly timbered and ornamented houses of typical Renaissance baroque design which surrounded a square dominated by the towering twin spires of Nikolai Church.

Johannes Kaempfer, who was a schoolteacher as well as a minister, was eager for his son to receive every opportunity for a good education. He sent Engelbert to study Latin in Holland and then to grammar schools in Lüneburg, Hamburg, and Lübeck in Germany. For his higher education, Kaempfer turned east to that most powerful German state, Prussia, where educational opportunities were greater because she had been spared many of the miseries of the long war. In 1672, at the age of twenty-one, Kaempfer enrolled at Danzig. At the completion of his studies in the same year, he presented a dissertation, "Exercitatio politica de Majestatis divisione," which was especially appropriate for the period of the absolute monarchs, Louis XIV of France and Charles XI of Sweden. In 1673 he received the degree in philosophy at Kraków, one of the great medieval universities, and then after an interval in Toruń began the study of medicine and natural history at the Lutheran university at Königsberg, which had risen to importance after the Reformation.

The medicine Kaempfer studied was taught entirely as an academic discipline, with a strong emphasis on botany and natural history. As a student, Kaempfer developed a proficiency in languages which proved invaluable in his years as a scientific explorer; he knew French, Swedish, Portuguese, English, Aramaic, Dutch, Russian, and Polish, as well as the usual Greek and Latin.

Early in his career Kaempfer adopted the popular habit of carrying a pocket-sized *Stammbuch* in which he collected the signature and brief comments of important persons he met in his travels. This *Stammbuch*, which is deposited at the Landsbibliothek in Detmold, includes entries through 1694 in Aramaic, Georgian,

Persian, Turkish, Chinese, Siamese, Japanese, and the common European languages.

After Kraków, since there were few opportunities for further study in disrupted Germany, Kaempfer decided to continue at Uppsala, which was renowned for its excellence in the sciences. However, before going to Sweden he returned to Lemgo to visit his family. On October 24, 1680, his father wrote in the *Stammbuch:*

> come from battle always victorious.
> Thus   as
> live   now meritorious.

In the same month his brother Joachim, who shared Engelbert's artistic ability, added a color sketch of a voluptuous mermaid and the words of warning "Blanditiarum virus tantum est ut ante mors grandis dolor sentiatur" ("So great is the venom of lust that before death great suffering is endured").

Kaempfer studied for one year at Uppsala under the direction of the strong-willed Olof Rudbeck, also a son of the clergy. Rudbeck was a multitalented man and must have been a source of inspiration to a student who also had many interests and a diversity of talents. He was an ethnologist, an architect, an author, and a composer of music, as well as a physician, a botanist, and an anatomist. He established at Uppsala the first anatomical theater in Sweden after studying at Leiden. This theater is on the roof of the main university building and is unchanged today; the backs of the rows of benches are painted to resemble Doric, Ionic, and Corinthian columns—silent testimony to Rudbeck's interest in architecture—and a house which Rudbeck designed still stands on the campus, nearly three hundred years after it was built. Rudbeck was a scientific pioneer on lymphatic circulation. He was the first in a long line of eminent Swedish botanists, and he established the earliest botanical garden in Sweden. He eventually forsook science to write "Atlantis" (never published), in which he endeavored to affirm one of the lost Atlantis myths which claimed that the world originated in Sweden.

Rudbeck's is another of the many famous names that are included in Kaempfer's *Stammbuch*. On August 18, 1681, the great man wrote, "Invidia nobilitas virtute comes, [signed] O. Rudbeck, Professor of anatomy and botany" ("Envy and fame are the companions of excellence").

Another entry in the *Stammbuch*, written during the same period, indicates how favorably Kaempfer impressed the faculty at Uppsala: "The outstanding character, distinguished erudition and superior knowledge of the art of healing of Engelbert Kaempfer will always be remembered at Uppsala. These words are dedicated as a symbol of permanent friendship and recognize a person to whom I bestow my continued good-will. Peter Hoffwenig, Rector of the Faculty of Uppsala and Verelius, philologist."

Through an acquaintance, Samuel Pufendorf, professor of law at Lund, Kaempfer learned that King Charles XI was planning an embassy to Persia. Although Charles was not an educated man himself, he recognized the importance of learning and leaned on the advice of scholars, the foremost of which was Rudbeck. Kaempfer was first offered an appointment as court scholar, but he declined the luxuries of court life to become a scientific explorer. He was young, keen, and adventurous, and the excitement of the post as secretary to a Swedish embassy to Persia far outweighed any advantages that life in the court might have offered him at that time. The embassy was intended to establish trade with the shah and to encourage him to break with the Ottoman Porte. Sweden was eager to restore the foreign trade that had dwindled during her years as a major combatant in the Thirty Years' War.

The embassy, under the leadership of a Hollander, Ludwig Fabritius, left Stockholm on March 20, 1683, and was detained at the Russian border because of an amusing Russian sensitivity —Persia was listed ahead of Russia in the official travel documents. Two months were then spent in Russia negotiating for permission to develop a possible trade route from Persia through that country, since Holland, France, and Britain controlled the sea lanes across the Baltic. Kaempfer's diaries on Russia and their relationship to the history and culture of the country have been examined by Loewenson, a Russian scholar, and his judgment is that they are "equal to any of the most important foreign works of the period" (p. 661).

It was at this time that the wide range of Kaempfer's interests and his zeal for gathering information began to be manifest in his diaries. On July 11, 1683, members of the Swedish embassy had an audience with the czarina, Sophia, and her half-brother, later to become Peter the Great. The "exceedingly vivid and fascinating description given by Kaempfer of the ten-year-old Czar Peter . . . is quite exceptional" (*ibid.*, p. 663).

At times it seems that Kaempfer must have pilfered letters or raided personal files. He obtained a copy of a letter to Sophia from Peter and Ivan in which as skulking young men they complain bitterly of actions taken by her authority and on which they were not consulted (Sloane MS 3063, Adversaria, British Museum). Nor were Kaempfer's interests restricted to his immediate environment. He gathered extensive notes on eastern Siberia—an area which he never visited. Russian translations of the Psalms, the Lord's Prayer, the Creed, and the Ave Maria are included in his diaries. His notes were written in a curious mixture of Latin, German, and French, which was not uncommon in that period, and at times on just a scrap of paper. It is easy to visualize this avid and inquisitive observer snatching up any available piece of paper to record information in the words of whatever language first came to his mind. This curious mixture of languages is not restricted to Kaempfer's daily diaries; one of his manuscripts is entitled *Dictionaire für tout les verbes Turquesques cum vocabulario*—French, German, and Latin.

Ten months after the embassy departed from Stockholm they reached Persia and were detained at Baku on the Caspian Sea to await a summons to the throne of Ispahan. The *Stammbuch* has an entry in Arabic with a sketch of a lovely woman with Persian features but in a Western dress which combines the blue and gold colors of the Swedish flag. The exceedingly curious and energetic Kaempfer immediately began to study the culture, to collect specimens representing the natural history of the area, and to practice medicine. His diaries include detailed observations on a volcanic field, a boiling lake, the naphtha wells, the absence of

43

whirlpools in the Caspian Sea, the town of Baku, and the ruins of ancient cities—all these in a single month. It is difficult to understand how Kaempfer could accomplish so much in a twenty-four-hour day. He exemplifies the best German traits—meticulous attention to detail and a limitless capacity for hard work.

When the embassy reached Ispahan there was further opportunity to study Persia, since a malignant constellation in the heavens indicated to the court astrologers that it would be unwise for the shah to see foreigners at that time. Six months elapsed before an audience was finally granted.

During these months Kaempfer developed an enduring and rewarding friendship with Father Raphael du Mans, the prior of the Convent of the Capuchins at Ispahan. The prior had gained an excellent knowledge of the language and country during thirty years as interpreter at the Persian court, and he passed along a great deal of information about Persia to Kaempfer.

At the end of the mission Kaempfer again faced the question of whether to continue his explorations or to choose the easier life of physician and scholar: "Germany was as yet engaged in war with the Ottoman Porte and the most Christian King when the Swedish Embassy, which I had the opportunity to attend as Secretary, was dismissed by the Persian Court. . . . I chose rather to lead the restless life of a Traveller than by coming home to subject myself to a share in the train of calamities my native country was involved in. Therefore, I took my leave of the Ambassador and his retinue with a firm resolution to spend some years longer in seeing other Eastern courts, countries and nations" (1727, 1: viii).

There were several opportunities for Kaempfer, including a post as physician to the court of the Georgian prince and a visit to Egypt. But the Capuchin priest Father du Mans encouraged him in his interest in the Far East, and Kaempfer entered the service of the Dutch East India Company, which had a trading station in Ispahan and whose ships were sailing the Persian Gulf. Thus for a second time Engelbert Kaempfer turned his back on the luxuries of court life to continue his fascinating but demanding life as a scientific explorer. On the advice of the captain of the

Dutch trade in Bandar Abbas, Herbert de Jaeger, he left for Bandar Abbas (Gombroon), a port at the head of the Strait of Ormuz on the Persian Gulf, in December, 1685, and here the perils of the explorer fell upon him. Bandar Abbas, a humid, unsanitary desert entrepôt where caravans and ships converged, was crowded with Arabs, Africans, French, Persians, Armenians, Indians, Dutch, and English—all eager for trade. In this miserable spot Kaempfer fell ill with a malignant fever which was followed by dropsy and then malaria; for a time he despaired of his life. His depression was deepened by the refusal of his superior, van Heuvel, to let him leave Bandar Abbas. However, friends finally interceded and he moved into the hills, where he eventually recovered. He continued to practice medicine and to study and record Persian culture until June, 1688, when he boarded an East Indiaman under the command of Vice Admiral Wibrand Lykochthon. The friendly letters from Father du Mans and Lykochthon at the British Museum indicate that Kaempfer's personality and enthusiasm as a scholar fostered a coterie of admiring relationships.

His diaries on Ispahan and the Persian Gulf area have extensive daily entries and vivid sketches—one of a bullock working at a Persian wheel and another of Ispahan from a distance, showing the minarets in excellent proportions and detail (Sloane MSS 2912, 3060, and 2923, British Museum). Representative essays from this period again demonstrate the breadth of Kaempfer's interests: descriptions of the Persian Court, the towers of Ispahan, *Dracunculus* infestation, the flood-broken mosaics of Persepolis, a bezoar, and the history of the date palm.

After departing from Bandar Abbas the fleet made a leisurely cruise toward the Far East, touching at Dutch stations in Arabia Felix, Malabar, Ceylon, Bengal, and Sumatra, and reached Batavia in September, 1689. From this journey we have the medical essays *Andrum*, an endemic hydrocele of Malabar; *Perical*, large swollen ulcers of the feet, peculiar to the people of Malabar; *Intoxicating Drugs of India and Persia;* and *The History of Asafoetida.* The essay on perical represents the first description of the edematous syndrome, ulcerated foot, known as mycetoma or Madura foot.

In Java, Kaempfer studied the botany of the island, which had already been extensively catalogued by the Dutch. Again he attracted the interest of his seniors, who in this instance encouraged him to study Japan and gave him much information about the islands. Two of them were former *opperhoofden* at Deshima: Johannes Camphuijs, now the governor general of Java, and Andreas Cleyer. Camphuijs "did much to assist . . . Kaempfer who borrowed his description of Japan in part from Camphuijs himself, the latter having often been on Dejima" (Blok, p. 526). (Undoubtedly Kaempfer was a glutton for information, but it is doubtful that he relied on Camphuijs any more than on other informants when he wrote his great book.) The third man was Herbert de Jaeger, whom Kaempfer had first met at Ispahan. De Jaeger urged him to collect maps, coins, books, and papers and to send them back to Batavia as Ten Rhijne had done (Sloane MS 3064, fols. 15–16 and 50–52). On May 7, 1690, Kaempfer's ship left Batavia and proceeded to Siam, where with characteristic dedication Kaempfer recorded an extensive description of the capital—Ayudhya—the land, and the people.

Kaempfer's ship, *De Waelstroom*, entered Nagasaki Bay on September 26, 1690, after several monsoons had so badly damaged the ship that the captain and passengers had determined to rest and provision in China and then return to Batavia. However, Kaempfer had in his possession a journal describing an earlier voyage to Japan which, despite the September monsoon, had ended safely in Nagasaki Bay. With this assurance, and by reminding the skipper of his probable punishment for the water-soaked cargo, Kaempfer persuaded him to hold his course for Japan.

The severe restrictions of life at Deshima, his inability to speak Japanese, and the un-co-operative attitude of the interpreters on his arrival did not daunt Kaempfer's thirst for knowledge of Japan. Soon his resourcefulness and knowledge began to reap dividends: "Liberally assisting them, as I did, with my advice and medicines, with what information I was able to give them in Astronomy and Mathematicks, and with a cordial and plentiful supply of European liquors . . . there was none that ever refused to give me all the information he could" (Kaempfer, 1727, 1:ii–

iii). Since the Japanese have a notoriously low threshold for alcohol, and Kaempfer with his German background and Dutch experience could hold his liquor, he had a hidden asset: he could drink, listen, and remember. An additional source of information was a "discreet young man, by whose means I was richly supplied with whatever notice I wanted concerning the affairs of Japan" (*ibid.*). Soon after Kaempfer's arrival this "discreet young man" had been appointed to be instructed by him in "physick and surgery" and to be his servant. With Kaempfer's advice he successfully treated the chief Japanese officer at Deshima and as a reward was permitted to spend two years with Kaempfer, learning to read and write Dutch, to study medicine, and, most important, to serve as a constant source of information, both verbal and written.

Kaempfer's assessment of Japanese medicine and surgery was that surgery was little developed and that the Japanese were ignorant of the "red hot irons, cutting knives," and other surgical instruments used by European doctors. He found the Japanese "more expert in physick than surgery—at least than European surgery" (*ibid.*, vol. 2, app., p. 63), and he respected their therapeutics since they preferred "gentler caustics than the West" and did not "load their patients with medicine" (*ibid.*, app., p. 35).

As an example of oriental theories on the etiology of disease, the cause of *senki*—a violent diarrhea—was "not at all in a morbific matter lodged in the cavity of the guts, which, they say, would occasion but a very slight pain but that the seat of it is in the membranous substance of some other part of the abdomen, as for instance of the muscles, the peritonaeum, the omentum, the mesentery, or the guts, and that by stagnating there it turns into a vapour, or rather into a very sharp sower spirit, as they express themselves, which distends, cuts and corrodes the membranes wherein it is lodged" (*ibid.*, p. 588).

The therapeutic potential of the hot springs with which Japan abounds impressed Kaempfer greatly, and he was distressed that their value was not more fully exploited. He believed that patients with venereal disease would profit by using them for a longer period. An amusing note concerns the use to which Buddhist monks put the hot springs on their temple grounds. The monks had assigned names to the springs, identifying some as purgatories for beer and sake brewers, others for cooks and wranglers, and still others for members of similar low trades. By promising to save the wayfarers representing these trades from such torrid fates, the monks were able to extract large sums of money from these gullible individuals.

Several of Kaempfer's entries are amusing and indicate that he possessed a quiet sense of humor. During a visit to the shogun's court at Edo, he was asked to examine a priest who had a fresh ulcer on one of his shins. The ulcer was of no consequence: "I advised him, however, not to be too familiar with Sacki Beer, pretending to guess by his wound what I did upon much better ground by his red face and nose, that he was pretty much given to drinking, which made the Emperor and the whole court laugh" (*ibid.*).

One of the most interesting and eccentric of the Tokugawa shoguns, Tsunayoshi, was the ruler during Kaempfer's two years at Nagasaki. He had been born under the sign of the dog and as one indication of his subservience to astrology decreed that the beasts could run freely under royal patronage, like cows in traditional India. To kill a dog brought capital punishment, and after death dogs were buried in hallowed ground. Kaempfer recounts the story of two Japanese who were laboring up a steep mountain with the corpse of a dog when one of them complained bitterly about the weight of their burden. The second one replied that he should be thankful that the shogun had not been born under the sign of the horse.

Kaempfer had the good fortune to join the *hofreis* to Edo on two occasions, and his meticulous diaries make him the most widely quoted source on this unique type of journey. The embassy first left Nagasaki in mid-February, 1691, after elaborate preparations and the procurement of gifts for the courts at Edo and Kyoto. The gifts were subject to approval by the governor of Nagasaki, and Kaempfer records that the governor had earlier refused to permit the Hollanders to present two red fire engines which they had shipped in from Batavia. The frequency of severe fires, which devastated the flimsy Japanese cities, should have made the fire engines a most welcome gift.

48

The *opperhoofd* was carried in a norimon while the other Hollanders rode horseback, seated on wooden saddles. There was at least one Japanese interpreter for each Hollander, as well as several escorts, the exact number being determined by the Dutchman's rank. Kaempfer added to his luggage a large box from Java in which he secreted a mariner's compass for accurate measurements of the directions of roads, mountains, and rivers. The box also contained an empty inkpot, as a hiding place for botanical specimens that he hoped to gather on the trip.

Kaempfer was captivated by the Japanese fans that were decorated with accurate maps indicating distances and was disappointed that he was forbidden to acquire one. However, he was more fortunate with the flora of Japan; through secret cash rewards as well as free medical advice the Japanese became "extremely forward to communicate to me what uncommon plants they met with . . . themselves great lovers of plants" (*ibid.*, pp. 399–400).

The first five days of the trip were spent in crossing Kyūshū from Nagasaki to Kokura; from Kokura they sailed across the Shimonoseki Strait to Shimonoseki.

Kaempfer was impressed with the clean and neat roads, which were lined by fir trees and repeatedly swept with brooms. All dung was collected for fertilizer, and in rainy weather the roads were sprinkled with sand and in dry weather with water.

It was not uncommon for the Hollanders to meet the retinue of a *daimyō* coming from Edo. One included more than 20,000 retainers, and Kaempfer recorded a meticulous description of the retinue's organization, members, and equipment. As the *hofreis* crossed the boundaries of a fief, the prince whose territory they entered sent a nobleman from his court to greet and escort them and four Japanese footmen to file beside each Hollander. The crowds that thronged the highways retired to the adjoining fields, bowing to make way for the Hollanders and their retinue. The peasants not only bowed low but turned their backs as an indication that they were not worthy to be seen by these distinguished visitors. But despite these evidences of their prestige, the Hollanders were locked in the center section of an inn each night after doors and screens had been boarded up. Kaempfer compared one inn to a Westphalia smokehouse.

The multitudes of people on the highways surpassed any crowded road in Europe. There were many pilgrims going north to the Ise Shrine, the seat of Shinto traditions, while others sought purity by visiting a series of lesser shrines or temples. Still others were simply enjoying one of Japan's favorite national pastimes—travel.

The passage from Shimonoseki to Osaka through the lovely Inland Sea lasted for eight days. Osaka was not only a great trading center but was as well a leading city for pleasure and entertainment. Kaempfer found the streets crowded with jugglers, performers, and mountebanks, and numerous theatrical performances were offered in public theaters as well as in private residences. He noted that the best Japanese sake was brewed near Osaka and that it was not only sold across the empire but also exported by the Dutch and the Chinese.

"Japan, the bawdy house of China" was the appellation used by Kaempfer because of the "unnumerable houses of prostitution that lined the highways" (*ibid.*, p. 439). Since prostitution was forbidden in China, the worldly pleasures offered by Japan were enjoyed by the many Chinese sailors who came to Nagasaki. Singing nuns who bared their breasts and begged were such pleasant company that Kaempfer dug into his pockets to keep one by his side for several hours.

Each village that the *hofreis* passed through had a public announcement board which listed the edicts against the Roman Catholics, as well as a posthouse and a public execution ground.

The Hollanders began each day's journey at dawn and continued until dusk and Kaempfer found the daily trip very long and tiring. Yet he had the dedication to spend many hours recording his observations as he rode along on a wooden saddle and when he was boarded up in an inn at night.

Beautiful Kyoto with its green mountains and numerous temples and shrines impressed Kaempfer deeply. Here the travelers presented gifts to representatives of the emperor and were taken to view art treasures. Kaempfer faithfully records 3,893 Buddhist temples, 2,127 Shinto shrines, 52,169 priests, 477,577 laymen, and 138,779 houses in Kyoto. He was impressed with the fact that in almost every house some kind of manufacture was under way— weaving, painting, carving, sewing, and lacquering.

The famed Tōkaidō road between Kyoto and Edo was even more crowded than the previous thoroughfares. Each *ri* from Nihonbashi (Nippon Bridge) in Edo was marked by a man-made mound on top of which a small tree had been planted. When he first saw Mount Fuji, Kaempfer noted that it was probably unsurpassed in beauty. Several large rivers fed by mountain springs crossed the Tōkaidō road and at times were so high and swift that to try to ford them was hazardous. Specially trained men who knew every hole in the river carried them across at a fee quite logically determined by the height of the torrent. If a traveler was lost or drowned, the man who had carried him was promptly put to death.

The importance placed on the purity of air and its relationship to disease is emphasized by Kaempfer's entries regarding a village near Edo, the air of which was cold, moist, heavy, and unhealthy. Camphuijs, one of Kaempfer's patrons at Batavia, later attributed his poor health to having passed through this village on the *hofreis*.

As the embassy approached Edo all of their baggage was meticulously probed and searched by police representing the shogun. The military ruler was always on guard against any possible insurrection by a *daimyō*, and every retinue was searched, especially for the two signs of impending revolt: those approaching Edo were searched for guns; those leaving were searched for women since wives would be spirited away from a scene of future hostilities. (Guns up and women down!)

Although they were forbidden to see anyone before the audience with the shogun, one of the court physicians came to Kaempfer seeking advice on the treatment of a patient. On the appointed day, which was always the last day of the second month on the Japanese calendar, the travelers were received by the shogun, who required the *opperhoofd* to approach by crawling on his hands and knees. Afterwards "we were ask'd a thousand ridiculous and impertinent questions" (*ibid.*, p. 534). For Kaempfer the questions included the diseases that he considered the most difficult

51

and dangerous to cure, his treatment of internal "cancerous tumors and imposthumations," and whether European physicians were seeking drugs to bring immortality, and, if so, had they made any progress (*ibid.*). In reply to the last questions, Kaempfer recommended Professor Sylvius' *Sal volatile Oleosum Sylvij*. When asked for a supply he responded that it could not be made in Japan but was available at Batavia. The shogun immediately directed that a supply be brought to Japan on the next ship. Kaempfer was required to dance and added a love song, but his keen eyes did not miss the opportunity to study the first lady of the court, who was secluded by a screen: "she was of a brown and beautiful complexion, with black European eyes, full of fire, and from the proportion of the head, which was pretty large, I judg'd her to be a tall woman and about 36 years of age" (*ibid.*, p. 532). He also remembered and recorded the ten courses served at a court dinner, including the varieties of food, their contents, color, taste, and the decorations at the table.

The only extant suggestion of a picture of Kaempfer appears in his sketch of the entourage winding along a road. One figure is designated as the doctor, but his features are not discernible.

Despite the bans against foreigners acquiring any materials on Japan, Kaempfer smuggled out manuscripts on history, geography, poetry, and religion as well as a dictionary, an almanac, maps measuring four feet, and many botanical specimens.

The prison-like existence at Deshima, the overbearing demeanor of the Japanese officials, and the cunning of the interpreters did not affect Kaempfer's impression of the Japanese and of the true state of the country. In an essay appended to his *History of Japan* he considers the desirability of opening Japan to the world and concludes that it had never been, "in a happier condition than it now is, governed by an arbitrary monarch, shut up, and kept from all commerce and communications with foreign nations" (*ibid.*, p. 75).

Kaempfer sailed from Nagasaki in November, 1692, and after a brief visit to Batavia and several weeks at Cape Colony returned to Amsterdam in October, 1693. He had spent ten years as a scientific explorer and now was eager to study and publish his observations. In Amsterdam he established an enduring friendship with the family of Johannes Parvé, especially the son Daniel.

At Leiden in April, 1694, at the age of forty-two, Kaempfer presented his doctoral thesis, "Disputatio Medica Inauguralis Exhibens Decadem Observationum Exoticarum," which included ten essays representative of his studies in the Middle East, India, and Japan.*

The award of the doctorate closed the most satisfying period of Kaempfer's life. Henceforth he was in a sense a tragic figure, a frustrated scholar with an overwhelming practice of medicine in his hometown, Lemgo. His superb studies on Russia, Persia, and Japan indicated that he was a man who belonged on the faculty at Leiden or one of the German universities. Yet he returned to Lemgo because of characteristic German dedication to the family land at Steinhaus near Lemgo and to accept the appointment as physician to the prince of Lippe at Detmold. His plans for early preparation and publication of his journals were thwarted, and it was not until 1712 that the first of these, generally known as *Amoenitates Exoticae*, appeared.† In the first fascicle there is a description of the Persian court. In the second there are essays on the absence of whirlpools in the Caspian Sea; Okesia, a peninsula in Médéa; the towers of Ispahan; the flood-broken mosaics of Persia; charts of Japan; and an account of the closure of Japan. The third fascicle includes a variety of essays on such subjects as acupuncture, moxibustion, asafetida, dancing snakes of the East Indies, and a history of Japanese tea. The fourth discusses the historical and botanical relations of the date palm of the

---

* I. De Agno Scytica, seu fructu Borometz; II. De Amaritie Caspii Maris; III. De Mumia Nativa Persica; IV. De Torpedine Sinus Persici; V. De Dsjerenang, id est, Sanguine Draconis, ex fructibus Palma Conifera spinosa elicito; VI. De Dracunculo Persarum; VII. De Andrum, endemia Malabarorum Hydrocele; VIII. De Perical, indigena Malabaris Hypersarcosi ulcerosa Pedum; IX. De Curatione Colicae per Acupuncturam, Japonensibus usitata; and X. De Moxa, Materia Cauteriorum apud Chinenses Japoniosque usitata.

† The full title is *Amoenitatum Exoticarum. Politico-Physico-Medicarum. Fasciculi V, Quibus continentur Variae Relationes, Observationes et Descriptiones Rerum Persicarum et Ulterioris Asiae.*

Persian crescent. The fifth fascicle describes Japanese plants worthy of the attention of travelers to the kingdom and includes the names of the plants in Chinese characters.

At the age of fifty-one Kaempfer married a sixteen-year-old girl whose anticipated wealth he relied on to free him from his obligations to practice medicine. The marriage was a tragedy; the bride was a shrew, and the three children born to her did not live. Kaempfer's frustrations were only accentuated by the discovery that she had only a small estate.

Engelbert Kaempfer died at Lemgo in 1716, when he was sixty-five years old, and he was buried at Nikolai Church. His life motto, *virtuti nihil invium* ("nothing is inaccessible to virtue"), was placed on his gravestone. Fortunately, he had completed the manuscript *The History of Japan* before his death. All of his manuscripts, diaries, and collections went to his nephew Dr. Johann Herman Kaempfer of Lemgo.

In the Preface to *Amoenitatum Exoticarum* Kaempfer mentioned that this was the "specimen" of three projected books: *Japan of Our Time; Herbarri Trans-Gangetic Specimen;* and a *Tripartite Travel Book*. Fortunately this statement came to the attention of Sir Hans Sloane of London. The over-all similarity of the lives of Kaempfer and Sloane is of such interest that it deserves recounting here. The two men were contemporaries but never met, nor did they correspond; both were versatile physicians, botanists, avid collectors, and keen observers. When Kaempfer was completing his studies of Japan, Hans Sloane was beginning a study of the natural history of Jamaica. While Kaempfer disappeared into the frustrating life of a practitioner in Westphalia, Sloane became the physician to British royalty, a man with a rich estate and great achievements.

Hans Sloane, the son of Scottish parents who had moved to Ireland, was raised in Ulster by the sea. At the age of nineteen he began to study medicine and botany in London and after four years went to Paris to study at La Charité Hospital and at the famed Jardin des Plantes. He received a "quick" medical doctorate in 1683 at a little-known medical faculty in the principality of Orange, just north of Avignon, since Protestants were not allowed to take degrees at French medical schools.

As a student and protégé of the famed Thomas Sydenham, Sloane soon became a busy practitioner in London and was elected to the Royal Society in 1684 and to the Royal College of Physicians in 1687. He undertook a voyage to Jamaica partly to justify his membership in these societies and partly to study native drugs. With commendable energy he collected more than seven hundred botanical specimens in Jamaica and with an artist developed an excellent set of drawings of the trees, flowers, and plants of Jamaica, as well as of the fish found there. As a shrewd Scotsman he purchased a large stock of Jesuits' bark, and the returns from its sale, added to the income from a large practice and the estate of a wealthy widow whom he married, made him a man of great wealth.

Sloane returned to Britain to become a physician of such note that his patients included the nobility and royalty—Queen Anne, George I, and George II. The first volume of *The Natural History of Jamaica* was published in 1707, but because Sloane was so busy the second did not appear until 1725. He was elected president of the Royal Society to succeed Sir Isaac Newton in 1727.

It was fashionable to develop "cabinets" or "collections" in this period and, because of his deep interest in natural history and his international circle of scientific acquaintances, Sir Hans Sloane became a leading collector. When he decided to acquire the Kaempfer collection and manuscripts he had two "agents" operating on the continent. One, a Hanoverian, Steigerthal, was the personal physician to George II.

In the Sloane collection there is a receipt in French signed by Johann Herman Kaempfer at Hanover in 1723 which acknowledges the payment by Dr. George Steigerthal of 450 *ecus* ("crowns"), approximately £80, for certain articles. The first purchase included the manuscript of *The History of Japan*, and Johann Caspar Scheuchzer of Zurich, who was Sloane's librarian, made the translation. The book, in two volumes, was published in 1727 under the imprimatur of Sir Hans Sloane as president of the Royal Society. Sloane continued to negotiate with Johann Kaempfer for the purchase of the remainder of the collection. It was the case of a canny Scot against a stubborn Dutchman. Kaempfer suggested that Sloane should make the price of the second purchase more attractive than that of the first. But Sloane was unyielding and after exchanges of correspondence the Scotsman was the victor. Sloane finally bought the lot for 112 crowns, just over £22 sterling. The total price of the two purchases was £102.

When Sir Hans died, at the age of ninety-three, it was found that he had determined to will his collections to the British people —for the sum of £20,000. He had reckoned they were worth at least £80,000 and had directed his executors that if Britain did not purchase the collections they should be offered successively to the science academies of St. Petersburg, Paris, Berlin, and Madrid—in all of which he held membership—on similar terms. Parliament enacted a bill to raise the necessary funds by a lottery, and the £100,000 that resulted permitted not only the purchase of the collection but also the founding of the British Museum, which was opened on January 15, 1759, just six years after Sir Hans's death.

Thus Engelbert Kaempfer's voluminous notes and sketches and his specimens from the natural history of Russia, Persia, Malabar, Ceylon, Java, Siam, Japan, and Cape Colony became one of the founding collections of the British Museum. The notes, manuscripts, and sketches are available there today. The botanical specimens were moved to the Museum of Natural History at Kensington. The specimens included Rhododendron, Ginko, Magnolia, Azalea, Bamboo, Gardenia, Cryptomeria, Clematis, and Aconite. The dried botanical specimens in the first of the two volumes, "although often small, are unusually good and in excellent preservation. This is one of the most important volumes in the Herbarium. . . . Probably no volume of the Sloane Herbarium has been more consulted. . . . The specimens have been much studied and variously identified" (Dandy, pp. 144–45). The second volume contains a number of scraps and is of little interest. Perhaps the seeds that germinated when the collections were hit by Nazi bombs, and when the resulting fires were doused with water, were from Kaempfer's materials.

The History of Japan is the most thorough compilation of information on the culture of Japan during the Tokugawa shogunate. Its publication was made possible by a truly international program: the studies of Japan by a German, serving the flag of The Netherlands, first translated by a Swiss who was librarian for a Scotsman born in Ireland who was one of England's leading physicians and citizens.

The original manuscript will probably never be published. Few books were being published in Germany when it was completed, and the Scheuchzer translation in English later came to be considered a better source than the original German. French translations were published at The Hague in 1729 and at Amsterdam in 1732. One year later, in 1733, a Dutch translation was published at Amsterdam, and in 1777, fifty years after the first publication, a German translation appeared, published at Kaempfer's home town, Lemgo.

Naturally the book found its way to Japan. In 1782 the lord of Hirado obtained a copy at Nagasaki, and this was later deposited in the Edo Observatory. Shizuki Tadao (1758–1806) translated into Japanese the essay on the desirability of Japan's continuing to be closed to the rest of the world.

Kaempfer brought one of the earliest, if not the first, collection of Japanese books to Europe—they have been described as probably the first Japanese books ever to be seen in Britain. In the Introduction to *The History of Japan*, Scheuchzer lists about sixty books and maps collected by Kaempfer. The volumes available at the British Museum today "represent a fair cross-section of the kind of literature that was generally current in Japan towards the end of the seventeenth century" (Gardner, p. 76). They include fiction, historical and legal works, guide and travel books, but there are no medical texts.

By all odds the most dazzling items in the Kaempfer collection at the British Museum are the stunning multicolored Chinese wood-block prints. The enthusiasm for Chinese culture in the Genroku period, which we have alluded to, was exploited by Chinese merchants who lived in a quarter near Deshima. Basil Gray has pointed out that, because of this proximity of the Chinese quarter to Deshima, it would not have been difficult for Kaempfer to acquire Chinese wood-block prints. With his botanist's eye, Kaempfer would have been attracted to the beautiful blossoms in the prints.

The first books illustrated with multicolored wood blocks were printed in China in 1606, at the end of the Ming dynasty. The principal centers for the production of the prints were Nanking, Hangchow, and Soochow in the Yangtze coastal region. Gray believes that all of the Kaempfer prints were produced at Soochow by Ting Liang-hsien and Ting Ying Tsung during the early K'ang-hsi period, 1662. The verse on one print reads: "Lotus flowers and lotus leaves filling a basket—the delicate beauty of a few blossoms of the tender lotus." On a second wood block the verse is "These round-clustered forms might be made of jade from the mountains of Ch'u—their radiance mirrors the bliss of wedded women" (Gray, p. 23).

Lemgo today is a thriving agricultural center of twenty-five thousand; the shining baroque public buildings and residences seem unchanged from the days when Lemgo was a booming town of the Hanseatic League. The twin spires of Nikolai Church are visible to the traveler several miles from the city. There is no marker to show where Kaempfer lies buried, but behind the church is the small house with a high gabled roof where he was born. It is used now as a storehouse and will soon be torn down. In the public museum there is a Kaempfer room with copies of *The History of Japan* and reproductions of his sketches. Across from the Nikolai Church is an inn which advertises that it was the home of Engelbert Kaempfer when he practiced in Lemgo, but this has not been proved. The visitor who is interested in Kaempfer may have the good fortune to meet the delightful scholar Dr. Karl Meier-Lemgo, Germany's leading authority on Kaempfer, and to be taken on a tour of the historic landmarks of Lemgo.

Engelbert Kaempfer has been called "the first German explorer" (Meier-Lemgo, 1960, p. i), "the Humboldt of the seventeenth century" (Ōtori, p. 29), and "the scientific discoverer of Japan" (Falkmann, p. 62). He richly deserves these accolades.

CHAPTER

III

Opening the Door to Western Medicine:
Carl Pieter Thunberg

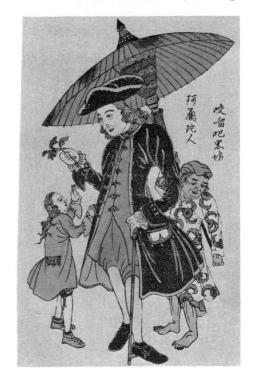

A FTER THE DEPARTURE of Engelbert Kaempfer in 1692, there
was a vacuum of scholarship at Deshima for more than
eighty years. The major developments in the eighteenth century
were on the Japanese side. A wise shogun set the door to Western
studies ajar, and a small band of Japanese scholars who were
eager to acquire knowledge from the West set the stage for the
rise of Western medicine.

The mental torpor of the physicians and barber-surgeons at
Deshima reflected the situation at home in The Netherlands.
The power of the Dutch as an overseas empire was entering a
period of decline: "the old pushing power of efficiency and
energy began to deteriorate. The rich citizens had had such an
easy life, generation after generation, that their wealth was
entirely taken for granted and, therefore, for that very reason,
slowly started to slip away from them" (Schöffer, p. 79). As the
eighteenth century progressed, the "old pushing power" referred
to by Schöffer dwindled steadily.

Deshima was no longer a lucrative trading post but had become instead an increasing drain on the coffers of the Dutch
East India Company. After 1672 the trade between the Hollanders and the Japanese at Nagasaki was tightly controlled by
the Japanese government, and the advantages previously enjoyed
by the Dutch in open trade sank steadily. All prices were set by
the Japanese government, and in 1715 items most valued by the
Hollanders—gold, silver, and silks—were barred, as were military
charts and maps, weapons, portraits of the emperor, and obscene
pictures. In the following year trade was tightened further when
the number of ships from Batavia involved in the annual trade
was limited to two.

Although the feudal rule of the Tokugawa shogunate seemed
on the surface omnipotent and omniscient, forces were afoot that
would eventually crumble the power. One of these was the
ascendancy of a merchant class with an advanced commercial
economy. By ranking the merchants in the lowest strata of feudal
society, below the peasants and craftsmen, the rulers had hoped
to build upon the dominance of a samurai warrior class based on
an agrarian economy. But the samurai and the lords became increasingly in debt to the merchants. The agrarian economy was

60

shaken by the heavy taxes laid on the farmers which with repeated ravages of famine and epidemic diseases precipitated agrarian riots.

Probably the first Japanese of national distinction to express the view that the empire should establish relations with the outside world was Arai Hakuseki (1675–1725), the son of a samurai. Hakuseki, the most versatile and distinguished scholar of his day, was designated by the shogun in 1711 to interview a Sicilian secular priest, Giovanni Battista Sidotti. The priest had entered Japan secretly in 1708 and was imprisoned at Nagasaki and later at Edo. Based on information that he gathered from his interviews with Sidotti and from conversations with the Hollanders at Nagasaki, in 1713 Hakuseki published *Seiyō Kibun* [Report of the Occident].* The three volumes include a history of the Sidotti affair and the prisoner's discussions of science, especially of the astronomy, history, and geography of European countries. The importance of the Arai Hakuseki–Sidotti relationship is that Hakuseki was an unofficial but highly trusted adviser of the shogun Iyenobu. Hakuseki was sufficiently impressed with Western learning to recommend that the seclusion policy be relaxed. As a sign of his interest in Western relationships he also recommended that Sidotti be freed and permitted to return to Europe. Neither recommendation was implemented; Sidotti died in Japan and the seclusion policy continued unaltered.

The first major step on the Japanese side to open the door to Western medicine was taken personally by the shogun Tokugawa Yoshimune, who ruled from 1716 to 1745. Yoshimune, the great-grandson of Tokugawa Ieyasu, is often ranked next to Ieyasu as the greatest of the fifteen Tokugawa shoguns. He applied zeal and imagination to such major programs as increasing food production, lightening the burden of the peasants, and reforming the *bakufu*, the legal system, and the role and activities of the great lords.

Yoshimune's contribution to the rise of Western medicine began with the Japanese calendar, that instrument which in China and Japan controlled a variety of events ranging from certain

* *Transactions of the Asiatic Society of Japan* 9(1881) contains a translation by the Reverend W. B. Wright of a major part of *Seiyō Kibun*.

responsibilities of the ruler to weddings and the planting of crops. It was the duty of the ruler to make available to his people a correct calendar, and Yoshimune found that the Japanese calendar was unreliable. He sought the advice of a Kyoto silversmith, Nakane Jouemon Genkei, who informed him that access to the Chinese translations of Western texts on astronomy and mathematics which had been banned was essential to any effort to correct the Japanese calendar. On this advice Yoshimune in 1720 directed that eleven books, all of which were Chinese translations of European astronomy texts, and books that did not contain information on Christian teachings, could be imported and circulated.

Yoshimune did not hesitate to look westward for assistance in expanding agriculture and food production. In 1723, at his direction, the Dutch imported Western horses, seeds, food, and birds. He also took steps to assure an adequate supply of medicine for his people in case the Dutch ships were unable to come to Nagasaki. On August 17, 1721, he ordered that a garden for the cultivation of medicinal plants should be established at Edo. An official physician, Ogawa Shōsen, was appointed director of the garden, which adjoined a hospital, Yōjōsho. When the Dutch ships arrived at Deshima in August, 1725, they carried eighteen varieties of medicinal plants primarily for the garden at Edo.

Twenty years after Yoshimune relaxed the ban on books he gave official sanction to the study of Dutch. He commissioned a forty-seven-year-old court physician, Noro Genjō, to study Dutch medicine and the *bakufu* librarian, Aoki Konyō, to study Dutch. In 1740 Noro Genjō and Aoki Konyō (also known as Bunzō) began their studies. Aoki Konyō had drawn Yoshimune's attention when after a severe famine he recommended the introduction of the sweet potato as a supplement to the minimal supplies of fish available to the citizens.

Noro Genjō had spent ten years at Kyoto studying medicine and botany. With this background his studies on Western drugs progressed more rapidly than the difficult and tedious task of compiling a dictionary assigned to Aoki Konyō. In 1741 Noro published an atlas of Dutch plants, *Oranda Honzō wake* [Explanation of Dutch plants in Japanese]. Twenty-three plants were described with their Dutch, Latin, Chinese, and Japanese names as well as their preparation and uses as medicinal agents. Five years later he published *Oranda honzō*, in which he described seven varieties of Dutch plants.

Aoki Konyō went to Nagasaki to study Dutch, and his news of the changing attitudes in the shogunate stimulated the interpreters: "When Aoki Konyō visited Nagasaki they insisted that he ask permission for them to read Dutch books and the shogun granted it promptly" (Krieger, p. 35).* In 1745 Aoki's influence at court was instrumental in obtaining official permission for three of the interpreters—Nishi Zenzaburō, Yoshio Kouemon, and Motoki Jindayu—to read and translate Dutch books. Aoki published an incomplete Dutch-Japanese lexicon in 1758, seven years after Yoshimune's death. In the words of Sansom, "It was naturally imperfect, but it was the herald of a growing interest in Western ideas, an interest which soon spread over the whole country" (1963, p. 170).

It was impossible for Japanese physicians to understand Western medicine as long as human dissection was banned. As in China, the strict laws forbidding dissection were based primarily upon reverence for the human body.

In A.D. 458 rumors were circulated in Japan that Princess Takuhata had committed suicide because of an unwanted pregnancy. To allay any suspicions an autopsy was performed under imperial writ, and the princess's virtue was confirmed by the fact that only a stone and a sac of water could be demonstrated.

The old Chinese book *Reisu* states that "the dead body should be dissected and observed" (translated from Nishi, p. 57). That this custom was followed in Japan is suggested in one of the haiku-style humorous but somewhat vulgar Senryū poems of the Edo period: "When a doctor prepares a globe-fish for cooking he is as careful as if he were dissecting a human body."† In another Senryū poem there is evidence that the Japanese dissected animals as well as human bodies: "A man dissected a goat and was sur-

---

* It is debatable, however, whether Aoki Konyō ever studied at Nagasaki.

† Globe-fish, or *fugu*, is a popular delicacy, but since the ovaries and the liver contain a highly toxic tetrodotoxin they must be removed with great care; otherwise a lethal poisoning will develop.

prised to find a love letter from a Maruyama geisha girl in its intestines."

The occasional dissections that were permitted in Japan were designed solely to confirm the theories of anatomy held in *Kampō* and were always performed on beheaded criminals. Since the Japanese could not defile themselves by handling a corpse, the dismemberments (they were not really dissections) were performed by members of the outcaste society, the *eta*, who were made responsible for the slaughtering of cattle and therefore were disdained by the other citizens.

The *eta* were willing to perform dissections in part because they could collect and dispense human bile, which was considered to be a potent medication for a variety of disorders, including intestinal cramps, a prevalent complaint. They were totally untrained in medicine, and their procedure was simply to cut out and exhibit the viscera, always in agreement with the anatomical theories of *Kampō*.

Until the sixteenth century, European anatomy was in a state similar to that of Japan and China. Ackerknecht has pointed out that "the anatomical illustrations of the Middle Ages are sadly similar to Chinese anatomical illustrations. The same speculative character and low quality mark them both" (1955, p. 83). Bodies were rarely examined in Europe and, as with the *eta* in Japan, the actual dismemberment was performed by a menial while the professor sat aloof on an elevated platform and pointed out from afar the structures as they were exposed. The dissection of the corpse of an executed criminal was ordained once a year as the *anatomia publica*. After the thirteenth century, dissections were practiced increasingly in Europe, especially under the eyes of the Church in Italy. The deficiency in European anatomical studies in the Middle Ages was that the doctors who supervised dissections saw only what they had learned from Galen.

The founder of modern anatomy was Andreas Vesalius (1514–64), who became professor of anatomy at Padua at the age of twenty-three. Five years later, in 1543, he published his great work, *De humani corporis fabrica*, in which he accurately described the anatomy of the human body and discredited the theories of Galen. Although Vesalius' findings were sharply attacked by the

Galenists, we can say that modern anatomy began in Europe two centuries before the pioneering efforts of a Japanese physician, Yamawaki Tōyō (1705–62) in Kyoto.

Yamawaki Tōyō was a paradox. On the one hand, he was the first Japanese to try to record an accurate description of the anatomy of the human body. On the other hand, he was an adherent and teacher of the *Kohō* (also *Kohōka*) school of medical thought, which forcefully advocated the renaissance of an ancient Chinese therapeusis based on sweating, vomiting, and purging. The *Kohō* school emerged in the seventeenth century under the leadership of Nagoya Geni as a reactionary movement against the *Ri-shū* school of Tashiro Sanki and Manase Dōsan (see Chapter I). Yamawaki Tōyō belonged to the second generation of the *Kohō* school and had studied under Gotō Konzan. Yamawaki placed great emphasis on the direct observation of facts—in the manner of the developments in Western medicine.

For the guidance of his students Yamawaki wrote *Yōjuin Isoku* [*Yōjuin* medical rules], which set forth the precepts of the *Kohō* school and his attitude as a teacher:

1. As a rule, the doctors should treat patients with the three therapeutic principles, that is to say, sweating, vomiting and purging. The aim of the study of medicine is to learn these three principles.

2. Pupils must learn the doctrines of their teacher. This is a principle of study.

3. Adopt the principle of the KOHŌ SCHOOL! It must be the way of present medicine. The KOHŌ SCHOOL is the basis of medicine; the present practice of medicine thus deviates from so-called orthodox medicine.

4. The way of the KOHŌ SCHOOL varies according to periods and regions, but diseases are unchangeable. We find the way of the KOHŌ SCHOOL through the diseases, if we will. Now is the best time for restoration of the KOHŌ SCHOOL.

5. We realize the fact that everything has its own properties, such as they are, and we collect these various things into one, so that the universe is formed.

6. Trivial healing arts should not be disregarded; there are reasons for their existence.

65

7. I take the position of the KOHŌ SCHOOL.

8. You may think that you cannot study the KOHŌ SCHOOL on account of its antiquity. But we still have clues which will allow us to study the KOHŌ SCHOOL.

9. The KOHŌ SCHOOL is now prospering. I intend to take the position of the KOHŌ SCHOOL with my family and followers.

10. It may be thought to be a reactionary tendency that we should put the KOHŌ SCHOOL into practice, but the fact is that the KOHŌ SCHOOL is the basis of medicine. Any SCHOOL is improved by practice.*

The opportunity for Yamawaki Tōyō to observe a dissection came through Kosuki Genteki, Hara Shōan, and Itō Yūshin, who were private physicians to Sakai Tademachi, *daimyō* of the Ohama clan in Wakasa and also the *shoshidai* for Kyoto. There is no evidence why they sought permission from the *shoshidai* to attend the dissection of a beheaded criminal. But we can speculate that they were stimulated to this interest by Yamawaki Tōyō and that they shared his discontent with the existing teachings and practices of medicine.

The dissection was performed by an *eta* on February 7, 1754, attended by Yamawaki, Kosuki, Hara, and Itō. A German anatomy text by Johann Vesling, *Syntagma Anatomicum*, is believed to have been in the possession of Yamawaki at the time of the dissection. In 1759 he published his observations in *Zōshi* [Description of the organs], which, although it contained many mistakes, was the beginning of experimental anatomy in Japan. The reaction of the entrenched practitioners of *Kampō* was best expressed by Sano Yasusada: "Dead organs have no function; the shape of organs is unimportant; only the living spirit is important" (quoted in Reinhardt, p. 17).

Yamawaki Tōyō's major contribution was to stimulate a spirit of investigation at a time when there was a mounting interest in foreign learning. This spirit came to full fruition fifteen years later with the monumental translation of a German anatomical text by a group of Edo physicians.

* William O. Reinhardt provided me with this translation by personal communication in 1964.

Soon after the dissection observed by Yamawaki, one of his students, Kuriyama Kōan, performed two dissections of human cadavers, the first in 1758, and another, on a female cadaver, in the following year. The second autopsy is of more than passing interest because it resulted in the first reasonably accurate description of the female reproductive system. The source of the cadaver is interesting. The corpse was that of a seventeen-year-old girl who had assaulted and seriously injured her husband when he chided her for infidelity. Although her husband's wounds were not fatal, she was sentenced to be crucified, but in an act of penitence and humanitarianism she agreed to have her body dissected, for which her sentence was reduced one degree—she was beheaded!

At about this time two Japanese physicians assumed historic roles of leadership in the rise of Western medicine in Japan. Through their contributions as teachers of Dutch and Dutch medicine and their heroic translation of a Western anatomy text they opened a century which saw Western medicine gain supremacy in Japan. The dramatic circumstances attending the translation have drawn too much attention to that event and too little to the inspirational careers of Maeno Ryōtaku and Sugita Gempaku as teachers—of Maeno as a scholar and of Sugita as the ardent champion of Dutch studies. The two leaders were a study in contrasts, yet remarkably complementary. Maeno was an introspective, aesthetic man totally dedicated to scholarship. Sugita was an articulate, pragmatic physician who combined the pursuit of scholarship with an intense dedication to its propagation. Together they made a perfect team.

Maeno Ryōtaku (1733–1803) of Nakatsu fief was raised by an intelligent yet eccentric uncle who, as we shall see, passed along both of these characteristics to his ward. Maeno's interests ranged from foreign languages and science to the study of *hitoyogiri*, a style of indigenous music. From his first days as a student, his primary goal was to master European languages to a degree that he would be able to read all books about Europe. He therefore began the study of Dutch as a student of Aoki Konyō in Edo.

Sugita Gempaku (1738–1818) of Kohama fief at Wakasa, the son of a physician, was sent by his lord to study Western medicine

67

with an Edo member of the Nishi family of interpreters of Nagasaki. At Edo he met Maeno Ryōtaku and in 1768 they were among the handful of Japanese who during the *hofreis* visited the Hollanders to learn Western medicine. More interested in the clinical practices of Western medicine than Maeno, Sugita had traced some of the illustrations from the most popular European surgical book of that period, the *Chirurgie* of Lorenz Heister (1683–1758). * Heister was the outstanding German surgeon of the first half of the seventeenth century and a powerful force in elevating the standards for the education of surgeons in Europe. As a sign of the wide popularity of *Chirurgie* in Europe, there were, in addition to seven German editions, three in Latin, ten in English, and translations into Spanish, French, Italian, and Dutch. Heister's book held a special place with Dutch physicians because he had studied at both Leiden and Amsterdam and in 1708 had served as chief surgeon of the army of The Netherlands. The Dutch surgeon at Edo discussed with Sugita the procedures and the instruments that he had copied from the *Chirurgie*.

Their brief association with the Hollanders stirred Maeno and Sugita to a complete commitment to the study of Dutch medicine. Although Sugita temporarily turned aside, Maeno was undaunted when the leading interpreter and scholar of Dutch, Nishi Zenzaburō, urged them to abandon their plans. He reminded them that although he had studied Dutch for fifty years he still had only a very limited facility in the language. Nishi had undertaken the task of singlehandedly compiling a Dutch-Japanese dictionary from a Dutch dictionary by Peter Marin. He had reached only the letter "B" when he died, soon after his advice to Maeno and Sugita, and undoubtedly was expressing justifiable frustrations to them.

About 1770 Maeno obtained permission from his *daimyō* to go to Nagasaki to concentrate on the study of Dutch. Sugita at the same time began to practice medicine in the manner of the Hollanders in his home in Edo.

* The full title is *Chirurgie, in welcher alles was zur Wundarzney gehoeret nach der neussten und besten Art, gruendlich Abgehandelt und in vielen Kupfertafeln die neu erfundenen und dienlichsten Instrumente, nebst den bequemsten Handgriffen der chirurgischen Operationem und Bandagen deutlich vorgestellet werden* (Nürnberg, 1718).

On his journey to Nagasaki, Maeno, in another expression of dedication to scholarship, vowed to seek no worldly gain until he had completely mastered the study of Dutch. Symbolically, he made this vow at the Dazaifu Temmangu Shrine, near Fukuoka, to which the greatest scholar of Chinese literature of the ninth century, Sugawara Michizane, had been exiled from Kyoto through court intrigues. Maeno desired a dedication to Dutch studies comparable to Sugawara's dedication to Chinese studies, for before his exile Sugawara had devoted himself exclusively to studies for which he was posthumously deified. Today Sugawara is worshipped throughout Japan as the God of Literature, and today the Japanese will travel several hundred miles to the Temmangu shrines at Dazaifu and Osaka to pray for success in the furtherance of knowledge, especially on the dreaded university entrance examinations. As further evidence of his interest in learning Dutch, Maeno adopted the name Rankwa ("incarnation of Holland").

Maeno spent 100 days as a student of Dutch with the leading Nagasaki interpreters, Yoshio and Narabayashi. He learned six or seven hundred Dutch words and acquired a simple Dutch dictionary. He also obtained a copy of a Dutch translation, *Ontleedkundige Tafelen*, of a German anatomical atlas and text, *Anatomische Tabellen* (*Tabulae anatomicae in quibus corporis humani*), published in Danzig in 1722 by Johann Adam Kulmus (1689–1745) of Breslau. The Dutch translation was by a Leiden surgeon, Gerarrdus Dicten, and was published at Amsterdam in 1734. In Japan it was usually referred to as *Tafel Anatomia*. The full title was *Ontleedkundige Tafelen benevens de daartoe behoorende Afbeeldingen en Aanmerkingen, waarin het Samenstel des menschenlijken lichaams, en het gebruik van alle deszelfs Deelen afgebeelden geleerd word*. The *Anatomische Tabellen* was a fortunate choice. It can best be described as a concise introduction to anatomy, but it was especially appropriate for Sugita and Maeno because it contained lucid explanations of anatomy as well as a wealth of illustrations with explanatory legends. A more detailed and sophisticated text would have made the almost impossible task that lay ahead hopeless.

On his return journey from Nagasaki, Maeno stopped again at Dazaifu and reaffirmed his dedication: "Only on deep reflection

I decided to learn Dutch. I only did so to make use of it for the sake of my country but never to gain glory or for self interest. May the Gods be my witnesses" (Krieger, p. 58).

While Maeno studied in Nagasaki, Sugita developed a fortuitous friendship with Nakagawa Junan (1739–80). Nakagawa was a physician in the service of the *daimyō* of Ohama and a daily student of the Dutch during their visit to Edo. An interpreter loaned Nakagawa two Dutch books on anatomy with the hope that he would sell them. Nakagawa first scrutinized the illustrations carefully with Sugita, who had been waiting for just such an opportunity. Sugita recognized immediately that the illustrations showed the viscera in a totally different form and relationship than did the charts of *Kampō* and determined to acquire one of the copies. Since Sugita did not have sufficient funds, the *karō* ("councilor of the clan") made the purchase; the book was another copy of the *Tafel Anatomia* that had been acquired by Maeno. Maeno returned from Nagasaki and soon there was an opportunity for Sugita and Maeno to test their belief in the reliability of *Tafel Anatomia*. On March 3, 1771, a friend of Sugita's informed him that there would be a dissection of a corpse at the execution ground, Kotsugahara, near Asakusa in Edo, the following day. Sugita and Nakagawa were joined by Maeno at the dissection, which was performed by a ninety-year-old *eta* on the beheaded body of Aocha Baba ("Green Tea Hag"). Sugita and Maeno carried their copies of Kulmus with them and were soon struck by the inaccuracy of the standard Japanese anatomy text: "When Ryōtaku and I compared what we saw with the illustrations in the Dutch book, we discovered that everything was exactly as in the illustrations. The six lobes and two ears of the lung, and the three lobes on the right and four lobes on the left of the kidneys, such as were always described in the old books of medicine, were not so found. The position and shape of the intestines and the stomach were also quite unlike the old descriptions" (translated from Sugita, 1959, p. 67).

As they returned to their homes from the execution ground Sugita and Maeno determined to take on the seemingly impossible task of translating Kulmus and reproducing the illustrations. They saw such an undertaking as a true service to their country.

Nakagawa volunteered his services and shortly they were joined by Ishikawa Genjō (1754–1816) and Katsuragawa Hoshū (1751–1809). Katsuragawa, although a physician to the *bakufu*, did not hesitate to involve himself in foreign studies and later proved of tactical as well as scholarly value to the team. The only Dutch sources available were the six or seven hundred words of Dutch that Maeno had learned at Nagasaki and the crude vocabularies that he had acquired there. At times the translators could not use existing Japanese or Chinese terms but found it necessary to invent completely new expressions. They frequently spent many hours puzzling over a single word. Sugita and Maeno decided to make the translation into *Kambun* because it was the preferred language of Japanese scholars. They undertook the translation with national pride: "It was Gempaku's (Sugita's) intention to send the translation to China to make known to the world that in Japan they wanted to begin revising Chinese medicine" (Krieger, p. 61). The translation was rewritten at least eleven times before Maeno was satisfied.

As they approached the end of their labors, Sugita and Maeno recalled that in 1767 a little innocent book, *Oranda banashi*, also known as *Kōmō-dan* [Tales of Holland], by Gotō Rishun, had been confiscated and the plates destroyed by the police because the Dutch alphabet was included in the illustrations. Therefore, in 1773 Sugita published as a trial balloon a preliminary report of five pages, *Kaitai Yakuzu* [Short atlas of new anatomy]. As a further safeguard, in 1774 copies of the completed work, *Kaitai Shinsho*, were presented in advance to the *bakufu* by Katsuragawa and official sanction was obtained. The entire five volumes of the *Kaitai Shinsho*, with numerous plates, were released in August, 1774. It was a monumental accomplishment even though there were, of course, errors in translation and the footnotes in Kulmus had been omitted. In addition, the illustrations were prepared from wood-block prints, which could not reproduce the detail and clarity of the etchings in the Dutch edition.

It is clear that, as the translation proceeded, Maeno and his collaborators drew on several sources besides Kulmus of Breslau. Professor C. R. Boxer (1950) has made a detailed examination of the *Kaitai Shinsho* and points out that the title page, which is

71

decorated with figures of Adam and Eve, is from Valverde's *Vivae Imagines partium corporis humani aeris formis expressae* from an edition printed at Antwerp by Christopher Plantin in 1566 (reprinted in 1579) or from the Flemish edition of 1568. Most of the anatomical illustrations in the text are from Dicten's translation of Kulmus (1734). The last four woodcuts in the *Kaitai Shinsho*, which show the tendons of the hand and the foot, are from Godfried Bidloo's *Ontleding des Menschelycken lichaams* (Amsterdam, 1690) or from the Latin edition of that title, published in 1685.

The *Kaitai Shinsho* was "the first European work to be printed and published by Japanese in Japan and therefore a landmark" (Sansom, 1962, p. 204).

The *Kaitai Shinsho* was crucial for the advance of Western medicine because it showed that the anatomical theories from China were incorrect and that the rational basis of Western medicine and science was superior. Because it was made by a group of physicians, the translation drew further attention to medicine as the leading field of scholarship for Japanese who were interested in foreign learning; and since the translation was from a Dutch text, it focused on Dutch and Dutch studies as the media for foreign learning.

The name of Maeno Ryōtaku does not appear in the *Kaitai Shinsho*, for he remained faithful to the solemn vow that he had taken at Dazaifu on his trip to Nagasaki. To have permitted his name to be listed as an author would have violated his commitment to disdain any glory or self-interest until his studies of Dutch were completed.

The most important contribution of the publication of *Kaitai Shinsho* was that it drew attention to Maeno and Sugita as the leading teachers of Dutch studies in Japan. Soon, under their auspices, a small but intensely dedicated band of scholars gathered in Edo to open the era of *Rangaku* ("Dutch study") and the flowering of Western medicine.

Carl Pieter Thunberg

The epochal publication of the *Kaitai Shinsho* coincided with the arrival at Nagasaki of Carl Pieter Thunberg (1743–1828), a

Swedish scientific explorer, physician, and botanist in the mold of Engelbert Kaempfer. Thunberg introduced the science of botany to Japan. His diaries (1795–96) include valuable information on Japanese culture, the state of Japanese medicine, and the attitude of the Japanese toward Western learning at the close of the eighteenth century.

The first Swede to be cited in the history of Deshima came to Nagasaki more than one hundred years before Thunberg. He was Oloff Erichson Willman who served as steward to the *opperhoofd* from 1651 to 1652 and subsequently wrote one of the earliest Western manuscripts on Japan (1667).

Willman's manuscript is referred to in the Sloane letters at the British Museum. It was discovered at Stockholm by C. H. H. Zollman, who offered to purchase the manuscript for Sloane. The chapter headings listed by Zollman include the history, the geography, and the climate of Japan, as well as two subjects that were dear to the hearts of all foreign observers—"concubinage," and "how they cut up their bellies" (Sloane, 1725). There is no record that the manuscript was ever purchased by Sloane. After Willman many of his countrymen served in the fleets of the Dutch East India Company, but Thunberg is the only other Swede cited in the history of the intercourse between Japan and the West.

Thunberg had the good fortune to be one of the handful of intimate student-disciples of Carolus Linnaeus, the founder of modern botany. Both Linnaeus and Thunberg were born and reared in Smöland, one of Sweden's poorest provinces, where the harsh life and the lack of resources encouraged habits of hard work and personal responsibility in any youth who aspired to success. Thunberg was born at Jönköping on November 11, 1743.

Endowed with a magnetic personality and a unique capacity for arousing burning enthusiasm for science in his pupils, Linnaeus was, as well, devoted to scientific explorations. Having traveled extensively in Europe, he now sat in Uppsala with his students deployed around the world studying, collecting, and shipping specimens back to the master. They included Hasselquist, who later died in Smyrna, studying in the Middle East; Lofling in Spain and then South America; Solander with Cook

73

in the South Pacific; and Per Kalm, a Finn, who studied in North America for three years. Thus it was only natural that Thunberg in due course become a member of this far-flung botanical empire.

When Thunberg enrolled at Uppsala in 1761, the university was noted throughout Europe for its strong science faculty led by Linnaeus in botany and by Celsus and Bergmann in chemistry. Higher education, like many other aspects of Swedish culture, was strongly influenced by the German universities, and in the medical faculties natural history and botany were important subjects. Uppsala was a lovely university town, bisected by the rushing Fyrisan River and dominated by the royal castle on one hill and the towering twin spires of the great Dom cathedral. On the riverbank were the famous botanical gardens developed by Linnaeus. Thunberg was a diligent and highly successful student; the dissertation "*De venis absorbentibus*," which he presented to a panel presided over by Linnaeus in 1767, brought recognition by the faculty:

> *Paastantissimum Ornatissimung Dominum Carolum Petrum Thunberg Smolandum, Medicum ad prascriptum Regiarum Constitutionum Academicarum in linguis eruditis ac Philosophius Disciplinis, suo convenientibus proposito, vita minatum adsensu Facultatis Philosophica, admissum adprobatuma esse, nomine Amplissima facultatis testor, Uppsalis 18 Aprilis 1767* [I hereby declare in the name of the faculty, that the most distinguished and admirable Master Carl Pieter Thunberg of Smöland is a Doctor in compliance with the requirements of the Royal Academy for the learned languages and systems of philosophy, appointed for life by endorsement of the faculty of philosophy after the approval of the great faculty, Uppsala, 18 April, 1767.] [Thunberg, Thunbergiana, 1767].

In 1769 Thunberg was accepted as a candidate for the doctorate in medicine and the following year successfully defended his doctoral thesis "*De Ischiade*." His medical diploma was signed on June 15, 1772, by Carolus Linnaeus.

Eight fascinating years of study and exploration in Europe, Africa, and Asia were initiated for Thunberg when Linnaeus recommended him for the Kahre Scholarship, which supported study abroad. With the award of the scholarship, Thunberg followed the trail of many other European students of medicine to Paris, which was emerging as the world's leading center in clinical medicine and surgery. At Linnaeus' suggestion he first visited Amsterdam where, through his intelligence and personal charm, he established an enduring and rewarding friendship with Professor Nikolas Burmann and his son. They were physicians, botanists, and scientists, as well as personal friends of Linnaeus. Thunberg's ability to promptly classify unidentified minerals, insects, and plants from their large collection so impressed the Burmanns that they volunteered to obtain financial support from the States General for him to study and collect specimens at the Dutch colonies of Surinam (Dutch Guiana) or Cape Colony. The excellent recommendation that Linnaeus sent to the Burmanns shows how highly he regarded his former student:

> *Numquam certe eligere potuissetis praestantiorem Apostolum quam D. Thunberg qui certe est diligens, acutus, submissus et in studium ardebtissimus. Si vivat certe multa praestabit pro tota Historia naturali et ab eo habebitis etiam immortalem nominis gloriam* [You could not possibly choose any better apostle than Dr. Thunberg, who verily is diligent, intelligent, unassuming, and with a high dedication to research. If he is allowed to live, he will most certainly achieve much for the whole of natural history, and you will obtain immortal glory from his name] [Svedelius, 1944b, p. 32].

Thunberg enthusiastically accepted the Burmanns' offer, but they agreed that he should first have a period of study in the great medical and surgical clinics of Paris.

Thunberg's diary includes an interesting comparison of opportunities for medical scholarship in The Netherlands and Sweden. The Burmanns complained that the academic salaries in Amsterdam were so low that it was necessary for them to divert their energies from scholarly pursuits to the financial advantages of the practice of medicine. Thunberg secretly congratulated himself that this was not a problem of the Swedish professors, who received adequate compensation from the universities and could devote their entire energies to scholarship.

When Thunberg arrived in Paris, that city's fame as the world's leading medical center was based on practical clinical teaching through the study of patients, excellence in physical diagnosis, and the meticulous study of disease at the autopsy table. The basic medical sciences, which received little emphasis, were appropriately termed "accessory sciences." In contrast, Thunberg's teachers at Uppsala placed strong emphasis on natural history and the lecture, with relatively little attention to practical teaching through patients. The French system deeply impressed Thunberg. "At Paris there is the most considerable medical college in Europe. . . . no other place affords so many opportunities for improvement in this science. . . . Theory is always accompanied and illustrated by practice. . . . the apparatus and methods of teaching all these sciences are as various as excellent" (Thunberg, 1795, 1:39).

Thunberg recorded extensive descriptions of the educational system, medical practices, and great teaching hospitals in Paris. Three thousand students were enrolled in the study of medicine and, with many others, Thunberg stood in queues for an hour or more to find a seat at the lectures of the most popular professors. Guards were posted in the lecture halls to preserve dignity, to assure that no student entered bearing arms, and to collect a small fee from each student. The final examinations were conducted in public by a tribunal of six professors who heard the student present his dissertation and then voted secretly with white or black balls. Despite the solemnity of the ceremony, a student rarely failed.

At the great old Hotel Dieu in the shadow of the Notre Dame, male patients were attended by friars and female patients by nuns. And once a month the servants of God passed slowly through the hospital in solemn but ominous procession carrying tapers and chanting liturgies. Fulminating disease was widespread; adults often lay two, and children four, in a bed. Patients frequently sickened and died before their families were aware of their illness, and it was necessary to display the corpses in a sidewalk exhibit so that relatives searching for loved ones might identify them.

Thunberg found special pleasure in the opportunities to study botany by attending lectures and examining specimens at the famed Jardin des Plantes. After nine months in Paris he returned to Amsterdam to find that his destination was now fixed as Japan.

The Burmanns and a group of wealthy merchants in Amsterdam and Haarlem were eager to support an expedition to collect the first major exhibit of Japanese botanical specimens for Holland. They had obtained a commission as surgeon extraordinary in the Dutch East India Company for Thunberg and had established quite adequate financial support for his studies. Because knowledge of Dutch was important for studies in Japan, they agreed with Thunberg that he should first spend some time at Cape Colony becoming more fluent in the language.

The voyage to Africa in the stinking, fetid ship filled with involuntary recruits who were too old, too sick, or too alcoholic to serve effectively as seamen was miserable. To add to Thunberg's frustrations in his repulsive environment, he was poisoned—and by the dominie! The latter was the caterer for the officers' mess and in a blunder issued white lead for the pancakes instead of flour! As a result, the captain, Thunberg, and the dominie—the latter serving an unwanted penance—were ill for two months with lead poisoning. Thunberg, always a prolific writer, later reported the nature and course of his illness to the Swedish Academy of Sciences.

Thunberg's visit to the Cape became far more than an intensive course in Dutch; he remained for three years studying botany, geography, ethnology, and linguistics. His collections and the descriptions of the flora of the Cape, published on his return to Sweden, earned him the title "The father of Cape Botany" (Svedelius, 1944b, p. 62). He prepared a vocabulary of the Hottentot language denoting dental, palatal, and guttural clicks for such words as tobacco, pipe, good day, dog, breast of a woman, and wolf. He made two expeditions into the hill country, which he called "Caffraria," and his observations are quoted today in descriptions of life at the Cape.

On May 18, 1775, more than three and a half years after departing from Amsterdam, Thunberg's ship sailed into the harbor at Batavia. With a warm and friendly personality, an extensive knowledge of European science, and a lively mind, Thunberg quickly established himself as a member of the intellectual circle at Batavia. He enjoyed the discussions on oriental culture, geography, and languages and prepared a concise Malay dictionary.

77

He observed that the bloody diarrheas which occurred frequently in the hot and humid colony were attributed to "saline particles" in the drinking water and that these were purportedly removed by plunging red-hot irons into the water. The Dutch East India Company realized a handsome profit from the sale of opium, a drug used widely by the Javanese, who "then go raving on the streets to kill men and the cry is 'Amok' and anyone can kill him" (Thunberg, 1795, 2:286).

In Batavia there were separate hospitals for the Dutch, Muslims, and Chinese. The latter had established a large community with characteristics that would fit any group of overseas Chinese today:

> The Chinese are reckoned the most numerous of all the strangers. They retain their national character, customs, and manners, are the most industrious people in the whole country, and indefatigable in everything they undertake. . . . The gardens about the town are chiefly taken care of by the Chinese. . . . They likewise farm the arrack distilleries, are skilled in almost every handicraft business, carry on an extensive commerce, cultivate the sugar cane, coffee, and indigo and—in short—are indispensably necessary [*ibid.*, pp. 266–67].

The attention to detail which characterized Thunberg's life was evident in the acquisitions he made before sailing for Nagasaki: "By way of preparing for my intended voyage to Japan, bespoke several necessary articles relative to my apparel, some of silk and others of cloth, with lace and other decorations of dress, in order that I might exhibit myself with propriety among the Japanese, who view the Europeans with greater attention than any other natural philosopher can examine the most rare and uncommon animal" (*ibid.*, p. 316). His ship dropped anchor off Deshima on August 17, 1775.

As an amusing anecdote, Thunberg recalls that the appearance of the ship's captain when he came ashore was strikingly different from that of his predecessors. For many years the captain had worn a special, voluminous robe when he left the ship; beneath its folds were strapped hundreds of guldens worth of contraband and other items for direct sale. The weight of the smuggled goods was frequently so great that the captain had to be supported on each side for navigational purposes. When this became obvious to officials of the Dutch East India Company, the special robe was banned. The Japanese were shocked to note that rather suddenly the captain, instead of appearing as a behemoth, had assumed the dimensions of other Hollanders.

For Thunberg, whose first love was botany, Japan was a treasure chest of botanical splendor. Then, as today, the magnificent gardens of flowers, plants, and trees indicated the Japanese love for horticulture. There was no other country where the delicacy and beauty of flowers, trees, and plants were as appreciated and enjoyed. Even by the humblest Japanese abode in a densely crowded community, the residents would find money to cultivate a few flowers or shrubs to impart a trace of verdure. Within the homes fresh flowers or shrubs or carefully arranged branches from bushes or trees decorated the *tokonoma*. The *kakemono* hung in the *tokonoma* displayed a seasonal bloom such as cherry blossoms in the spring and chrysanthemums or red maple leaves in the autumn. Women peddling flowers from carts loaded with blooms went from house to house throughout the year.

Thunberg was so eager to begin his botanical studies that even confinement at Deshima could not thwart him. His first specimens were collected by sifting the fodder that the Japanese brought for the livestock. He soon developed a second source of specimens by encouraging "the interpreters, whom I daily instructed in medicine and surgery, to gather the leaves, flowers, and seeds of all plants that they could find" (*ibid.*, 3:37). Japanese doctors who came to learn Dutch medicine also brought native plants as well as minerals and drugs for his collection. The collection grew so rapidly that when the East Indiamen returned to Batavia at the end of their trading missions they carried many botanical specimens destined for the Burmanns in Amsterdam.

The interpreters were now an invaluable source of information and materials. In the eighty-five years since Kaempfer had complained bitterly about their hostility, relationships had improved greatly, and Dutch had completely supplanted Portuguese as the language for communication. The interpreters enjoyed the financial returns as well as the status value of their knowledge of Dutch medicine, and a number of them had large and profitable medical practices. "They are obliged to apply themselves particularly to the study of physick and are the only persons in the country who practice this art after the European manner, and with European remedies which they can easily procure from the Dutch doctors" (*ibid.*, p. 34). But the interpreters continued to rely heavily on the advice of Thunberg, who had "frequent opportunities of serving them and their sick relations, friends and dependents, by good advice and well-chosen medicines" (*ibid.*, p. 35).

When he was permitted to botanize in Nagasaki, Thunberg observed many people, particularly the aged, with inflamed, weeping eyes. He attributed this condition to atmospheric pollution. The "stench arising from the urine and ordure as also from the offals of the kitchen . . . was frequently in hot weather so strong and insupportable, that no plug introduced into the nose could dispute the passage with it and no perfumes were sufficient entirely to disperse it" (*ibid.*, p. 144).

Thunberg's diaries include a number of interesting notes on Japanese medicine. Acute diarrheal disease (*senki*), as described by Kaempfer (1727, vol. 2, app. 3, p. 29), continued to be prevalent. Thunberg, reflecting the humoral theories on the causation of disease, attributed its high incidence as well as that of rheumatism to intense daytime heat and sudden gusts of wind. The Japanese physicians placed the primary blame on overindulgence in sake, which they stated would close the pores and prevent perspiration. The paroxysms of *senki* were at times so violent that male patients were left with a hernia. Japanese physicians believed that *senki* was best treated with acupuncture; nine needles were inserted over the stomach. Smallpox was common, but Japanese physicians had no knowledge of the use of vaccination. Venereal disease was as frequent as diarrhea, and the only medical treatment was the use of "decoctions to purify the blood" (Thunberg, 1795, 3:79). Later, Thunberg introduced Japanese physicians to the use of mercury, then the most effective agent in the therapy for syphilis. Scrofula, with glands as large as a man's fist, was seen frequently.

In general the impact of Western medicine on Japan had been small: "their Physicians have no insight into Anatomy and

Physiology and are very little acquainted with the remedies which they prescribe. The only persons among them who have a little more knowledge of these are either the physicians of the Court, or the Dutch interpreters who have an opportunity of acquiring some degree of knowledge from the European physicians" (*ibid.*, pp. 73–74).

When he visited a patient as the consultant to a court physician, Thunberg was frustrated because he was not permitted to interrogate the patient directly or to examine him. A long curtain was drawn around the bed and the court physician relayed Thunberg's questions through the curtain. Medical practice fell into five categories: internal medicine, surgery, acupuncture, moxibustion, and massage. The practitioners of acupuncture roamed the streets at night proclaiming their skills. The practitioners of internal medicine had their heads entirely shaved; they relied on simple remedies, primarily decoctions containing either a diuretic or a sudorific. There continued to be a large import of medicine from China. Ginseng, moxa, and camphor were the most popular remedies, along with a number of native products from India and the Indies—the stinktree, serpent stones, and rhinoceros horn. Acupuncture and moxibustion were performed as frequently as phlebotomy in Europe—it seemed that everyone received moxa.

Thunberg recorded the most interesting description of the annual *hofreis* to Edo of any of the European doctors; it was, as for the other scientific explorers, the highlight of his service in Japan. By Japanese decree the retinue was required to leave Deshima on the fifteenth or sixteenth day of the first month of the Japanese calendar. The three Europeans—the captain, Thunberg, and the secretary—accompanied by two hundred Japanese, left the gate of Deshima on March 4, 1776. Their colleagues at Deshima and all the Japanese who worked on the island accompanied the entourage to the limits of Nagasaki where the Europeans entered a Shinto shrine and drank sake with traditional Japanese formality as a sign of the importance of the event. When they returned to the highway, "all these Japanese who were now to part with us, had placed themselves in groups, according to their different ranks and conditions of life, for above a half mile in length, on both sides of the road, along which we were travelling, which not only made a very fine appearance, but likewise did us great honor" (*ibid.*, p. 95).

The Japanese who had been designated by the governor of Nagasaki as the native leader of the expedition was carried in a large norimon in front of which marched a soldier bearing a tall pike as a symbol of authority. The chief interpreter served as treasurer for the expedition and paid all expenses for inns, food, ferries, tolls, and other items. The total cost to the Dutch was about sixty thousand guldens; Thunberg suspected with good reason that the chief interpreter turned a handsome personal profit from his position. The three Hollanders were carried in norimons, and Thunberg compared his relatively comfortable and protected vehicle with that of poor Kaempfer, who had been required to ride horseback at the mercy of the elements.

Thunberg was struck by the colorful appearance of the retinue.

> The whole of this numerous caravan, composed of different people, and travelling in such different ways, formed a delightful spectacle for an eye not used to similar sights, and was to us Europeans the more pleasing, as we were received everywhere with the same honours and respect as the princes of the land, and were besides so well guarded, that no harm could befall us, and at the same time so well attended, that we had no more care upon our minds than a suckling-child; the whole of our business consisting in eating and drinking, or in reading and writing for our own amusement, in sleeping, dressing ourselves and being carried about in our norimons [*ibid.*, pp. 99–100].

And he showed his familiarity with Kaempfer's great book: "In the year 1691, when Kaempfer went on the journey to the court, the ambassador took another route to Sinongi; viz, across the bay near Ōmura, to avoid which we took a round-about way to Isafaia, but without sailing across the large bay by Shimabara, which is the road that Kaempfer took, in the year 1692" (*ibid.*, p. 103). Thunberg's botanical eye was repeatedly captured by the countryside. When they reached an agricultural area he noted that "the country was cultivated all over . . . exhibiting the finest fields, loaded with rice and other grains" (*ibid.*). He seized every opportunity to collect botanical specimens and was frequently assisted by the Japanese. The physical stamina which he had acquired on his expeditions upcountry at Cape Colony now stood him in good stead; he was able to race up slopes and be well underway in gathering specimens before his Japanese escorts could catch up with him. Naturally, the Japanese were attracted by his enthusiasm for their country. When he admired a beautiful fir tree, the interpreters helped him to obtain seeds as well as young shoots from the tree. In turn they benefited from the stream of information on the trees, plants, and flowers that poured from Thunberg. He identified dozens of specimens: barberry bush, spiraea, japonica, iris, lily, viburnum, magnolia, clematis, azalea and many others. He noted in his diary that for sheer beauty the maples and gardenias of Japan could not be surpassed. The passage on the Inland Sea, with the boat hugging the shore, afforded an unusual opportunity to observe the beautiful trees and plants that lined the beaches. For Thunberg the countryside between Osaka and Kyoto could be matched only in Holland.

Familiar with the strict schedule imposed on the *hofreis*, patients lined the roadside in several areas to be treated by the doctor. They entered the Tōkaidō road at Sanjō Bridge in Kyoto and headed northeast. "Here as well as at the other places, were sick people, who had come from the adjacent parts for advice from the Dutch physician in their chronical complaints. These complaints were frequently either large indurated glands in the neck, and cancerous ulcers, or else venereal symptoms, which had generally taken too deep root" (*ibid.*, p. 143).

The weeks at Edo during the *hofreis* were intellectually delightful for Thunberg. He was surrounded day and night by enthusiastic and intelligent students. Their questions ranged over a wide spectrum of subjects—medicine, botany, astronomy, natural history, natural philosophy, and rural economy. The nature of their questions repeatedly indicated that they had acquired a beginning knowledge of Western science, and their enthusiasm and assiduousness proved that they were eager for more.

The importance of Western knowledge was now firmly planted in the minds of the leaders at the shogun's court: "Five physicians

83

and two astronomers were the very first who, after obtaining leave from the council of the empire, in a very ceremonious manner came to see us and testify their satisfaction at our arrival" (*ibid.*, p. 176). Astronomy was in great favor in Japan, but because of their limited knowledge of Western astronomy Japanese astronomers were unable to compose a perfect calendar. Two of the junior physicians from the shogun's court knew a little Dutch and through them the chief court physician asked Thunberg about the treatment of many common medical problems such as fractures, epistaxis, phimosis, hemorrhoids, furuncles, toothache, and ulcerated throat.

In the ensuing days the two junior court physicians came daily to study with Thunberg. One of them was Katsuragawa Hoshū, personal physician to the shogun, and he wore the hollyhock court insignia on his robes. The second, Nakagawa Junan, was physician to one of the leading feudal princes at his residence in Edo. Katsuragawa and Nakagawa were acquainted with the rudiments of Western botany, zoology, mineralogy, and natural history. With considerable pride they showed Thunberg copies of Dutch books on medicine and natural history—Johnston's *Historia Naturalis*, Lorenz Heister's *Chirurgie*, Woyt's *Treasury Gazophylacium*, and Dodonaeus' *Herbal*. (A copy of *Herbal* had been presented to the shogun by the *opperhoofd* a century earlier.) Katsuragawa and Nakagawa brought Thunberg many specimens of indigenous drugs, plants, and minerals. A special gift was a bezoar from a horse's stomach which they believed had secret medical potency.

The relationship between teacher and students was ideal. Thunberg referred to Katsuragawa and Nakagawa as his "much beloved pupils" who in turn "loved me from the bottom of the heart so as to regret greatly my departure" (*ibid.*, p. 206). As a symbol of his lasting affection he gave them the most prized possession of a European doctor, his silver spring lancet, and, at their request, he signed a certificate stating that he had instructed them in Western medicine.

The inability of the shogun to conceal his interest in foreigners produced an amusing sequence when he received the Dutch mission at his court. After the presentation of the annual report and the gifts, Thunberg and the other members of the embassy were shown through sections of the shogun's castle. A number of the princes bombarded them with questions and proudly displayed samples of Dutch writing. The Dutch soon recognized that one of the princes who was studying and interrogating them with special intensity was actually the shogun incognito!

When the mission departed for Nagasaki, Thunberg's luggage contained forbidden maps of Japan, Edo, Nagasaki, and Kyoto and a number of Japanese books. He was especially pleased with the botanical atlases that he acquired and considered the plates to be of such excellence that they would deserve singular commendation in Europe. Upon their arrival in Kyoto one of the mikado's personal physicians sought Thunberg's advice on the identification of a number of plants which were purported to have medicinal value. The Japanese guards were not as attentive on the return journey, and in Osaka Thunberg had no difficulty purchasing blooming bushes and shrubs which he carried back to Deshima. They arrived at Nagasaki on June 29, 1776.

Thunberg was so effective in his relationships with the Japanese that, as the end of his year approached, the *opperhoofd* became almost insistent that he remain for a second tour. Thunberg, however, decided to return to Uppsala. He doubted that he could make any further significant contribution to the advancement of Japanese science; he had a massive collection of specimens to classify, and he wished to enter an academic career. The boredom of his life of smoking, drinking, and dull conversation at Deshima was a source of discontent. On November 30, 1776, he sailed from Nagasaki.

When the ship reached Batavia Thunberg was saddened to find that a number of his friends had died from fevers. He then spent five months botanizing in the East Indies. On the homeward cruise there was a seven-month visit at the Dutch factory in Ceylon, during which Thunberg made two botanical expeditions to the Blue Mountains. The East Indiaman finally sailed into Amsterdam on October 1, 1778, its passage through the English Channel having been hazardous because a number of the crew were too weak to handle the lines. The avaricious captain and mate had sold the best of the crew's rations at Cape Colony; they were later placed on trial and dismissed from the service of the Dutch East India Company.

Thunberg could report to the Burmanns and to his sponsors that his mission had been accomplished. He had fulfilled their charge to collect specimens in Japan and had added the bonus of an extensive collection from Cape Colony. He felt particularly gratified when he saw that plants which he had shipped back from Asia and Africa were already blooming in Holland. In turn, Dutch scientists were so impressed with his accomplishments that they offered him a professorship, which he declined.

Before returning to Sweden, Thunberg visited London, primarily to study the Kaempfer collection. His host was another scientific explorer and botanist, Sir Joseph Banks, president of the Royal Society, who had sailed with James Cook to the South Seas and had acquired a collection that included plants from every part of the world. But Thunberg's interest was primarily in Japan: "Kaempfer's Manuscripts and Collections of Herbs, together with the Drawings and Designs, were the articles which gave me the greatest pleasure to see here" (*ibid.*, 4:290). On March 14, 1778, nine years after his departure to study for one year in Amsterdam and Paris, Thunberg returned from Europe, Asia, and Africa to Ufstad, Sweden.

While Kaempfer's return to Germany had led to a life of frustration, Thunberg's return to Sweden led to a life of academic achievement. Soon after his arrival he had an audience with King Gustav III, to whom he reported the major results of his studies and scientific explorations.

On March 5, 1781, Thunberg was appointed demonstrator in anatomy at Uppsala University; on November 7 of the same year he became extraordinary professor of anatomy; and on September 7, 1784, just six years after joining the faculty, he achieved the most honored appointment in the Swedish medical faculties, professor of medicine and botany at Uppsala. In the same year he was elected president of the Academy of Sciences in Stockholm. His rapid advancement rested in part on the steady stream of manuscripts which began soon after his arrival at Cape Colony and continued during his years at Batavia and Nagasaki. On his return he became an even more prodigious writer, with publications in Swedish journals and in the journals of Paris, Haarlem, London, and Berlin.

In 1784 Thunberg's most important scientific contribution, *Flora Japonica*, was published. It includes descriptions of more than seven hundred and fifty herbs and woody plants. The majority are flowering plants, phanerogams, and the remainder are cryptogams, non-flowering plants. The book is illustrated with many drawings.

Fauna Japonica was published in two parts in 1822–23 with Linnaean binomial nomenclature and descriptions of more than three hundred and thirty Japanese animals and insects. This was the first summary of Japanese fauna (Ueno, p. 85). Thunberg's studies on the East Indies were recorded in a thesis, *Florula Javanica*, published at Uppsala in 1825 (Thunberg, Winberg, and Widmark).

In addition to his responsibilities as a professor at Uppsala, Thunberg continued to be a long-distance teacher for his beloved students Katsuragawa and Nakagawa at Edo. Thirty-two of their letters to Thunberg are at Uppsala and they show that there was a lively exchange of books and botanical materials between Uppsala and Edo despite the Japanese "bans" against foreign intercourse. The ease with which scientific materials flowed between Japan and Sweden is clearly shown in a letter from Nakagawa Junan to Thunberg (see Thunberg, Thunbergiana):

My dear Carel Pieter Thunberg

I thank you who teaches herb and apothecary arts which sciences are from last year, also I thank you since I have received three copies of books you sent for Dr. J. Hoffman. With my lord servant Sijemon I will now send you 100 various seeds of plants and a few dried leaves. Following this I shall send you next year Japanese books if you write a letter saying what you want. I request two large dictionaries namely for Dutch and for Latin by Prof. Marin and also new improved apothecary books. I request you to write the prices of the above in a letter.

> Dr. Hossie thanks my Lords
> for his testimonies

> Your servant
> N. Zjunnan
> [Nakagawa Junan]

Edo, 11 March, 1777

The exchange of additional seeds of flowering plants was commented on in several other letters.

Thunberg did not restrict his attention to botany; he sent Katsuragawa and Nakagawa the basic specimens for a zoological collection and included instructions, chemicals, and other materials so that they might expand the collection with Japanese specimens. Kaempfer's *Amoenitates Exoticae* and his own *Flora Japonica* were included in the books that he sent to Edo.

Thunberg's voluminous and detailed reports on the botany of Japan and Cape Colony, especially the *Flora Japonica*, brought him distinction in scientific circles in Sweden and abroad. He was awarded honorary or corresponding membership in more than sixty learned societies, and his certificates of election to many of these are included in the Thunbergiana at the university library in Uppsala: Edinburgh, 1778; The Netherlands, 1785; the Royal Society, 1778; Switzerland, 1793; Florence, 1797, and the Linnaean Society at Paris, 1821. In return he sent duplicates from his Japanese, Cape Colony, Ceylonese, and Javanese collections to the British Museum and to gardens in Leiden, Geneva, Kiel, and other cities. He was highly respected in Russia and in 1802 declined one of the most distinguished scientific posts in that country, director of the botanical garden in the capital, St. Petersburg. But the Russians bore him no ill will, and three years later he was elected to the Society of Naturalists in Moscow. His greatest honor, happily, came from his own king when he was invested with the Order of the Vasa at the rank of commander in 1815.

The old Linnaean botanical gardens by the Fyrisan River were by now quite unsatisfactory; there was no space for expansion, the climate was damp, and they were heavily shaded. Thunberg persuaded King Gustav III to endorse the transfer of the gardens of the royal castle to the university to serve as the new botanical gardens. They were spacious, on high land adjoining the campus, and there was an opportunity to erect a suitable building to house the expanding collections, led by Thunberg's materials from Africa and Asia. In 1785 Thunberg, who never discarded a specimen or any other item that he had collected, deposited 15,050 species of plants mounted on 23,510 sheets; 6,000 shells;

and 25,000 specimens of insects mounted in 80 cabinets in the new museum. The morale and international prestige of Swedish botanists had plummeted when Linnaeus' widow sold his collections to Britain, and the massive deposition by Thunberg was a step in the restoration of national scientific pride.

In this period it was customary for a professor to write the doctoral theses for his students. These afforded another outlet for the information that Thunberg had amassed; their titles include "African Medicine," "The Iris," "The Gladiolus," "Expectorant Drugs," "Insects," "Poisonous Plants of Macassar," "Cinchona," "Belladonna," and, of course, "Moxibustion."

In due course Thunberg was elected rector magnificus at Uppsala, an essentially honorific post which passed to the more distinguished and senior professors. His residence was a pleasant farmhouse in Tunaborg on the outskirts of Uppsala where he spent his final years reviewing his collections and honors and playing cards. He died on August 8, 1828, at the age of eighty-five.

There are twenty-six large volumes in the Thunberg collection at Uppsala, of which six are on botany; the others include materia medica, ornithology, zoology, fauna from Cape Colony, and Thunberg's personal history.

One volume on materia medica contains an extensive list of prescriptions, including the ingredients for the *Sal volatile Oleosum Sylvij* which Kaempfer had recommended to the shogun to prolong life. There is a list of drugs that Thunberg found in the dispensary of the hospital at Batavia.

The second volume on materia medica lists a number of diseases and their therapy, beginning with "asthma, aphthous, arthritis, apoplexy, and dysmenorrhea." Peruvian bark and ipecac were recommended for the treatment of fevers; cinnabar, China bark, or Peruvian bark for epilepsy; balsam of Peru for gonorrhea; and mercury for syphilis.

The six volumes on botany are profusely illustrated with drawings of flowers including the aster, anemone, canna, peony, iris, viburnum, camellia, hibiscus, and verbena from Deshima.

Svedelius has described Thunberg as Linnaeus' foremost pupil, the most renowned botanical explorer of his age, and the greatest botanical collector. The first accolade is debatable; Thunberg was not a creative scientist and his achievements rest more on his diligence and capacity for hard work. Nordenskold cited Johan Christian Fabricius, a Dane, as perhaps the student who best understood Linnaeus' scientific methods and how to apply them in his own research. Linnaeus referred to Lofling, who studied in Spain and South America, as his most beloved pupil. Professor Sten Lindroth, who holds the Chair in the History of Science at Uppsala and has studied the members of the Swedish Academy of Sciences in the eighteenth century, states that Thunberg was not one of Linnaeus' most "interesting" students. Thunberg was satisfied with the spiritless tasks of collecting and describing as many fresh species as possible. His enthusiasm for collecting and describing, his warm and friendly personality, and his patience, were three attributes that made him so successful in Japan. In just one year he amassed an extensive collection which, through his European associates, was important in informing European scientists about Japan.

Carl Pieter Thunberg's position in the history of Western science in Japan is clearly recognized by the Japanese. In Nagasaki the Japanese Science Council and the Japanese Botanical Society have erected a monument with an appropriate inscription: *"Viri Optimi Doctissimque quo primus in Iaponiam Botaniam Importavit"* ("Of an excellent and very learned man who was the first to bring botany to Japan").

四

CHAPTER

IV

The Flowering of Western Medicine:
Philipp Franz Balthasar von Siebold

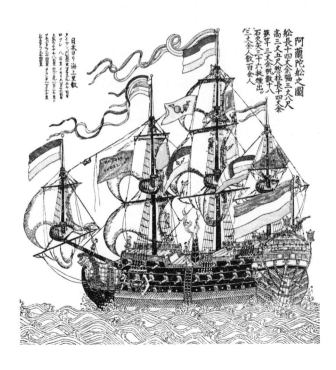

THE EMERGENCE OF Maeno Ryōtaku and Sugita Gempaku as teachers and champions of Western studies, coupled with the publication of *Kaitai Shinsho*, signaled an era of mounting Western influences. There was a striking forward thrust, not only in the study of medicine, but in other fields as well, including the Dutch language, natural history, astronomy, and mathematics. This period, which spanned the three-quarters of a century before the opening of Japan, is referred to as *Rangaku* ("Dutch study"), for a small band of progressive scholars, *Oranda* ("Holland"), replaced China as the repository of knowledge.

The remarkable rise in Western studies during *Rangaku* was made possible by an interesting fusion of indigenous intellectual growth with foreign scientific and technical achievements. The orderly life and absence of armed conflict that characterized the Tokugawa shogunate encouraged intellectual activity and the pursuit of inquiry. The *Rangakusha* ("Dutch study persons") were attracted by the rational, pragmatic basis of Western science and technology, which contrasted sharply with the traditional abstract Confucian philosophy that dominated the Japanese scene.

Rangaku was another period when the outward-looking Japanese—"the frog in the well"—borrowed and adopted intensively, as they had from China during the seventh, eighth, and ninth centuries. This outward look was in striking contrast to the inward concentration of the Chinese, who continued to disdain all foreign intellectual currency.

With the emergence of *Rangaku* the center for foreign studies moved from Nagasaki to Edo. It was a natural shift, for with a large community of scholars and artists, including calligraphers, poets, painters, wood-block artists, dramatists, musicians, and Confucian scholars, the shogun's capital had become the seat of the cultural and intellectual life of the empire. Further, the shift was symbolic because it brought the study of Western knowledge from the isolation of remote Nagasaki to the heart of Japan. Henceforth Nagasaki served primarily as the "postgraduate center" for the study of Dutch.

Eleven medical schools in which *Kampō* was the basis of instruction were opened under the sponsorship of the *bakufu*, or feudal lords, after the middle of the eighteenth century (see

TABLE 1

Medical Schools Teaching Traditional Medicine Sponsored
by *Bakufu* or Han, 1752–1852

1756 Saishunkan, opened by Lord Hosokawa Shigekata of
Kumamoto Han in Kumamoto.
1774 Igakuin, opened by Lord Shimazu in Kagoshima.
1785 Meihokan, opened by Tokuyama Han. After 1843 the program included both Western and Chinese medicine.
1789 Meitokukan, opened by Akita Han.
1791 Seijukan, taken over by the *bakufu;* the name was then
changed to Igakukan.
1792 Igakukan, opened by Kishū Han in Wakayama.
1801 Igakuryō, opened by Aizu Han.
1805 Saiseikan Igakujo, opened in Fukui.
1811 Igakukan, opened by Sendai Han.
1840 Nan'en Igakujo (or Kōseikan), opened in Hagi by Yama-
guchi Han; taught both Dutch and Chinese medicine.
1841 Kōdōkan, opened by Lord Tokugawa Nariaki of Mito
Han.

Table 1). But the striking development in this period was the
establishment of twelve private schools teaching Western medicine
in Edo, Kyoto, and Osaka (see Table 2). The first Shirandō, was
opened in Edo in 1786 by the greatest of the *Rangakusha*, Ōtsuki
Gentaku, also known as Bansui (1757–1827). An examination of
his career and his scholarship gives an illuminating picture of
the intellectual vigor of *Rangaku*.

The son of a physician trained in Dutch medicine and serving
in the Sendai domain, Ōtsuki, whose given name was Shigetada,
was apprenticed to another Sendai physician, Takebe Seian, at
the age of thirteen years. After nine years he was drawn to Edo
in 1779 by the fame of Sugita Gempaku and Maeno Ryōtaku,
with whom he studied medicine and Dutch. It was at this time,
according to Professor Numata Jirō, that he changed his name
to Gentaku—"as a combination of Gen from Gempaku and Taku
from Ryōtaku" (1961, p. 67). Sugita wrote of Ōtsuki: "I have
found that Gentaku is a practical man by nature. . . . he never

TABLE 2

Private Medical Schools That Taught Western Medicine,
and Their Founders

1786   Shirandō Juku, established by Ōtsuki Gentaku in Edo.
1801   Kyūridō Juku, established by Koishi Genshun in Kyoto.
1801   Shikandō Juku, established by Hashimoto Sōkichi in
        Osaka.
1805   —— Juku, established by Inamura Sanpaku in Kyoto.
1817(?) Shishisai Juku, established by Naka Ten'yu in Osaka.
1829   Nisshūdo Juku, established by Tsuboi Shindō in Edo.
1834   Shōsendō Juku, established by Itō Genboku in Edo.
1836(?) Chōzendo Juku, established by Kō Ryōsai in Osaka.
1838   Tekiteki-sai Juku, established by Ogata Kōan in Osaka.
1838   Wada Juku, established by Satō Taizen in Edo.
1839   Junsei Shoin Juku, established by Shingū Ryōtei in Kyoto.
1846   Taiseikan Juku, established by Narabayashi Sōken in
        Nagasaki.

Note: (?) indicates probable date of establishment of school.

talked of things he did not fully understand; he did not like super-
ficiality. I liked him because of his talent and taught him as well
as I could. In the end I entrusted him to Ryōtaku to guide him in
the study of Dutch science. As I thought, he was so industrious that
Ryōtaku soon laid a foundation of knowledge which enabled him
to understand Dutch books" (Krieger, pp. 73–74). Maeno quickly
recognized Ōtsuki's remarkable talents and dedication and made
him his prize pupil.

After six years in Edo, Ōtsuki went to Nagasaki where he
studied for one year with the leading teachers among the interpreters: Motoki Jindayū, Yoshio Kōsaku, and Shitsuki Tadao.
When he returned to Edo in 1786 he entered the practice of
medicine. But his first love was the life of a teacher and scholar,
and in the same year he opened Shirandō. Until Ōtsuki's death
forty-one years later, Shirandō was the leading center for Western
studies in Japan.

The variety of manuscripts that flowed from Ōtsuki Gentaku's
pen was remarkable. In 1783, four years after beginning the

serious study of Dutch, he began to write a language text for those who wished to study Dutch; it was published in 1788 as *Rangaku Kaitei* [Ladder to Dutch study]. In the introduction Ōtsuki acknowledged the ascendancy of Holland over China as the seat of knowledge: "Until now China was considered the most civilized country. Holland, however, is superior because next to literature, it possesses science" (*ibid.*, p. 79). He stated that the contributions from Holland included: "medicines, instruments, and books for studying astronomy, geographical topographical survey, and detailed and excellent medical books. These books give us the proper ideas on how to initiate our studies. We want to absorb the merits of their science, because they are dealing with the most important aspects of the human way of life" (translated from Numata, 1961, p. 111).

In the first volume of *Rangaku Kaitei*, Ōtsuki set forth a number of reasons for studying Dutch and traced the development of Dutch studies in Japan. The second and most important volume included instructions on how to read, write, study, pronounce, and translate Dutch. The significance of *Rangaku Kaitei* in the advancement of Western learning in Japan approaches that of *Kaitai Shinsho*. It was the first book written and printed by Japanese dealing exclusively with a Western language. Because it was written in the Japanese syllabary, *Katakana*, instead of *Kambun*, the Chinese characters used in most treatises, *Rangaku Kaitei* was of special value to young students and the average citizen.

In 1767 Sugita Gempaku had copied illustrations from Heister's *Chirurgie* and later started to translate a small section of the text. Ōtsuki Gentaku assumed the task and in 1790 published *Yōi Shinsho* [New book on surgery]. It soon became one of the most widely read and important medical books in Japan and played an essential role in the development of Western surgery. There are four volumes, profusely illustrated with drawings of scalpels, forceps, scissors, drains, sponges, and dressings.

In 1794 Ōtsuki recorded the discussions between the Hollanders and the Japanese at the time of the *hofreis* in *Seihin Taigo* [Talks with Western guests]. Of special significance was the fact that this was made possible by the sponsorship of the shogun's surgeon, Katsuragawa Hoshū, and Ōtsuki expressed his pride and his gratitude: "We owed it to Professor Katsuragawa's kind help that we could personally talk to the Dutch. But we owed it to the renown of our study that we, in spite of being small vassals, could talk to the guests of the Shōgun and question them. I mention this with deep emotion and joy to make this memorable fact immortal" (Krieger, p. 103).

Under the auspices of Kimura Kenkado, a wealthy sake distiller at Osaka whom he had visited on his trip to Nagasaki, Ōtsuki published in 1786 *Rokubutsu Shinshi* [New record of six things]. This contained a series of translations from Dutch on mermaids, the unicorn, nutmeg, mummy, saffron, and *Polyporus officinalis* (a fungus).

Ōtsuki continued his campaign to glorify Holland and Western culture instead of China through his association with the book *Kōmō Zatsuwa* [Red-hair miscellany], published in 1786, for which he prepared the prefatory note. The author, Morishima Chūryō, was the younger brother of Katsuragawa Hoshū and had been encouraged as a *Rangakusha* by Isaac Titsingh. To avoid the wrath of the *bakufu* for criticism of the Japanese and Chinese languages, Morishima Chūryō used the device of placing his thoughts in the mouths of Hollanders whom he and Ōtsuki purportedly had interviewed at Deshima. He derided the complexity of the thousands of characters in the Chinese language when twenty-six letters sufficed for foreign countries using the alphabet. Morishima praised the charitable institutions of the Dutch, especially the orphanages, which he contrasted with the widespread practice of infanticide in Japan.

Two years later, Ōtsuki's commitment to Western culture was again heralded in *Ransetsu Benwaku* [A clarification of misunderstandings in theories about the Dutch]. Here the author, Arima Genchō, reported a series of interviews with Ōtsuki in which the latter cited many admirable qualities of the Dutch. Ōtsuki dismissed the ridiculous notion that the Dutch raised their legs like dogs to urinate and similar false impressions that were current in Japan. He praised the Dutch system of medicine and the Dutch diet and included a brief but surprisingly accurate description of world geography illustrated by a map showing continents and many countries in proper relationship.

In 1798 Ōtsuki completed an expanded second edition of the *Kaitai Shinsho, Jūtei Kaitai Shinsho* [Revised new book of anatomy]. Sugita Gempaku had recognized that there were many errors in his original work and assigned the preparation of a corrected version to his most gifted student, Ōtsuki. After ten years Ōtsuki produced the new edition, in which he not only corrected Sugita's errors and omissions but added a great deal of information which represents about two-thirds of the book.

Other writings of Ōtsuki Gentaku demonstrate his wide range of knowledge and interests: a translation on syphilis, an introductory primer for the study of Dutch, several treatises on geography, and a monograph on gunnery.

With such a number and variety of publications it was only natural that in 1811 Ōtsuki Gentaku was appointed as the first staff member of the newly established *Ranshoyakkyoku*, or Office for the Translation of Dutch Books. Beyond the national recognition that this appointment brought Ōtsuki, it was also symbolic of the importance to the government in Edo of ready access to information on Europe. By establishing the bureau, the shogunate brought the compilation of such information under its direct control. The founding of the translation office also strengthened the status of Edo as the center of foreign studies in the land.

An interesting instance of Ōtsuki's total dedication to Dutch culture was his renunciation of the oriental lunar calendar and adoption of the solar calendar of the West for the celebration of Japan's most important holiday, *Shōgatsu* ("first month of the year"). Ōtsuki chose the first of January in contrast to the traditional Japanese lunar date and named his holiday *Oranda Shōgatsu* ("Dutch New Year"). At the first *Oranda Shōgatsu* in 1794, Ōtsuki convened his fellow-*Rangakusha* and gave initiative to the formation of a society of Dutch translators.

The celebration of Ōtsuki Gentaku's *Oranda Shōgatsu* is charmingly portrayed on a *kakemono* made by Ichikawa in January, 1794, which hangs in the library of Waseda University in Tokyo. It shows twenty-nine Japanese in *haori* and *hakama* kneeling in ceremonious manner on *tatami* mats around a large cloth on which the *Shōgatsu* banquet has been laid. The setting is traditional Japanese but the utensils on the table indicate that this was an

Oranda celebration. Instead of chopsticks, there are knives, forks, and spoons; instead of sake cups, there are European goblets. One of the guests is seated in a European chair wearing a Dutch uniform and smoking a long clay pipe like an old burgher in Amsterdam. A Japanese painting that may be of Hippocrates shows him adorned with a Dutch hat.

Although Ōtsuki Gentaku was firm in his conviction of the importance of *Rangaku* as a practical science, he did not wish to see it sweep away the rich Japanese traditions. As early as 1786 he wrote: "As to the government of the country and human relations, there have been emperors and we have had Shintoism since the ancient times. Individuals representing the upper and the lower classes have held deep respect for each other. Moreover, Confucianism has been so excellent and detailed that everyone tries to learn its teachings by heart and to obey them. There is no reason to expect Dutch learning to correct our deficiencies. However, if we compare medicine within and without the country, we can understand the superiority of the latter" (translated from Numata, 1961, p. 113). Ōtsuki sought a place for *Rangaku* within the fabric of the Japanese culture.

More than ninety students enrolled at Shirandō to study with Ōtsuki, and during his lifetime he had the satisfaction of seeing them establish schools for Western studies in Osaka and Kyoto as well as extend *Rangaku* in Edo. Hashimoto Sōkichi (1763–1836), who had earned a livelihood painting designs on parasols in Osaka, came to study at Shirandō at the age of thirty. In 1801 he opened a school, Shikandō, in Osaka where he taught Western medicine and Dutch. Some of Ōtsuki Gentaku's versatility is reflected in the range of Hashimoto's publications—in medicine, botany, electricity, and cartography. He repeated Benjamin Franklin's kite experiments and published a book on electricity, *Erekiteru Kyurigen* [Research on electricity]. Hashimoto has been accurately described as "the founder of Dutch studies in the Kansai area" (translated from Sekiuma, p. 65).

Another pupil of Ōtsuki Gentaku, Koishi Genshun (1742–1808), opened a medical school, Kyūridō, in the heart of the old capital city, Kyoto, in 1801. There were dormitory accommodations for only twenty students but, according to Sekiba Fujihiko, since the number of day students was not restricted, there were close to one thousand students registered at the school (*ibid.*). Therefore, a new name was added, *Ryūmon-rō* ("dragon-gate pavilion"), based on the Japanese legend that a carp may grow rapidly and emerge as a dragon. Not long after the founding of the school, Koishi Genshun was succeeded by his son, Koishi Genzui.

Although the *bakufu* gave official endorsement to Western surgery in 1793 with the appointment of Katsuragawa Hoshū, internal medicine progressed more slowly. There was little interest in the pathophysiology of disease. One of Ōtsuki's leading students, Udagawa Genzui (1755–97), published in 1792–93 *Seisetsu Naika Senyō* [Selected points of Western theories on internal medicine]. It was a translation from the Dutch version of Johannes de Gorter's *Medicinae Compendium* (Leiden, 1731), *Gezuiverde Geneeskonst, of Kort Onderwijs der Meester Inwendige Ziekten* (Amsterdam, 1744, 1762). Udagawa, who had been a practitioner of Chinese medicine, described how his contacts with Maeno, Sugita, Ōtsuki, and other *Rangakusha* had converted him to the study of Dutch medicine. He reserved special praise for Ōtsuki: "I love him as my brother and respect him as my teacher" (Krieger, p. 98). Udagawa's translation was the first comprehensive text on internal medicine to circulate in Japan and it served as a model for several subsequent texts: "Before Udagawa there were other advocates of internal medicine but their work only consisted of notes on what they had heard" (*ibid.*, p. 98).

One of the most brilliant of the *Rangakusha* was another convert from *Kampō*, Udagawa Genshin (1769–1834); his conversion was the work of Udagawa Genzui. Born in Ise Province as Yasuoka Genshin, he came to Edo in 1790 and was persuaded by Udagawa Genzui to study with Sugita Gempaku. However, the old master would not tolerate Genshin's mischievous conduct and finally expelled him. Genshin was salvaged for Western medicine by Genzui and then studied with him and with Ōtsuki Gentaku. It was a wise move, for Udagawa Genshin became a prolific writer; one of his books, *Seisetsu Ihan Teikō Shakugi* [General outline of medical precepts], 1805, was especially useful to the average practitioner of medicine. The *Ihan Teikō*, as it was popularly designated, was a three-volume manual of anatomy based on the European texts of Stephanus Blankaart, Jean Palfyn, and Jakob Benignus Winslow. Included in the manual were extensive anatomical descriptions and a comprehensive discussion of the physiology of digestion. Three years after publication of the *Ihan Teikō*, Genshin published a superb accompanying atlas under the sub-title *Naishō dōban-zu* [Inside form, copper plates]. This atlas was of historic as well as medical significance, for it contained the first copper plates to be used in Japan for a scientific atlas. For the student of anatomy the reproductions from the copper plates gave far greater clarity of anatomical details than had the woodblock prints used in previous texts. There were fifty-two prints in all, prepared by an Edo artist, Aōdō Denzen.

Udagawa Genshin may be described as the father of pharmacology in Japan because of his publication of four pharmacology texts. The most important of these was *Oranda Yakkyō* [Mirror of Dutch medicines], which was published in 1828. It was the first Japanese text that described European pharmacology, and was based on the dozen or more European pharmacology books then circulating in Japan.

The Udagawa dynasty continued to play a leading role in *Rangaku* through the person of the son-in-law of Udagawa Genshin, Udagawa Yōan (1798–1846). Of special significance to the rise of Western medicine in Japan was his contribution to the development of Linnaean botany. Thunberg had been the first to introduce European botany based on Linnaean principles, and Udagawa Yōan was the first to publish detailed descriptions of the Linnaean system: *Botanikyō* [Scriptures of botany], in 1822, and *Shokugaku Keigen* [Source of botanical knowledge], in 1834. Yōan emphasized that botany is a science which dissects the structure and analyzes the function of each part of a plant. He may be credited with initiating the scientific movement that replaced the old Chinese-based *honzo*, which simply gave the name of a plant and its medicinal properties, with dynamic botany. Thereby he played the leading role in placing studies of Japanese materia medica on a firm Western scientific basis.

The lack of a reliable comprehensive Dutch-Japanese dictionary was a major barrier to the advancement of *Rangaku* until the end of the eighteenth century. Earlier in that century a Nagasaki interpreter, Nishi Zenzaburō, began to prepare a dictionary based on Peter Marin's Dutch-French dictionary, *Woordenboek der Nederduitsche Fransche taalen: Dictionaire Flamand et Francais* (Amsterdam and Utrecht, 1729), but this was never finished. As we have noted, Aoki Konyō prepared an incomplete Dutch-Japanese lexicon in 1758. Maeno Ryōtaku assumed the work of Nishi Zenzaburō briefly, but he was soon diverted by other studies. At the suggestion of Ōtsuki Gentaku, one of his leading students, Inamura Sanpaku, joined a Nagasaki interpreter, Ishii Tsuneemon, in renewing the task, and they added a second important Dutch-French source book, *Nieuw Nederduitsch en Fransch Woordenboek* (Amsterdam, 1717), by François Halma, to the project. Subsequently they turned to a third source, a Dutch-Latin dictionary by S. Hannot, *Nieuw Woordenboek der Nederlandsche en Latynsche Taalen*, also published in Amsterdam. As the work progressed, Udagawa Genzui and Udagawa Genshin were added to the team. It was a Sisyphean task; the Dutch letters were printed, and the Japanese equivalents inscribed to the right, character by character, by Udagawa Genshin, for a total of 80,000 words in each of the thirty copies that were published. On February 18, 1796, with Inamura Sanpaku listed as the author, the thirty copies appeared under the title *Haruma wage;* it is frequently referred to as *Edo wage.* As Professor Numata Jirō has pointed out, the book was simply too voluminous to publish; one of the copies which is available today consists of nine volumes with 64,035 words listed on 2,187 pages (1961, p. 73).

In 1810 Fujibayashi Fuzan, who had studied with Inamura Sanpaku, selected the 27,000 most common words from *Haruma wage* and published 100 copies of a small dictionary, *Yaku-ken* [Translation key].

When the Napoleonic Wars ended the trade between Batavia and Nagasaki in the early nineteenth century, the scholarly *opperhoofd* Hendrik Doeff, with time on his hands and the assistance of several Nagasaki interpreters, prepared another Dutch-Japanese dictionary based on Halma's lexicon. *Nagasaki*, or *Dofu Haruma*, was not published until 1833, almost twenty years after

Doeff had left Deshima. This was used more widely than Inamura Sanpaku's *Haruma wage*.

The first English-Japanese dictionary, *Ageria Gorin Taisei*, was published in handwritten form in 1814; the first printed Japanese-English dictionary, *Waei Gorin Shūsei*, was published in Shanghai in 1867 by an American missionary, Dr. J. C. Hepburn.

One of the pioneering Japanese practitioners of Western surgery to gain a place in medical history was Hanaoka Seishū (1760–1836). He is reported to have performed a surgical operation in 1805 using as an anesthetic *mafutsusan*, which, according to Hideomi Tuge, was made from *Datura*, a genus of plants which includes the Jimson weed, *Datura stramonium*. In an illustration of this operation Hanaoka's surgical instruments are shown to include a lancet, scalpel, scissors, hammer, saw, and chisel. Another illustration sketches an operation and carries the legend "A drawing of an operation on breast cancer" (Tuge, p. 74).

A small group of leading Japanese physicians and surgeons now had available a substantial body of information on the principles of Western medicine. Their great deficiency was in the application of this knowledge to the diagnosis and treatment of disease. They needed to be taught the practice of medicine. Fortunately, in 1823 a remarkable young German physician and surgeon came to Deshima to spend six years in Japan, and one of his principal activities was to teach clinical medicine. He was the most versatile of the European physicians who came to Deshima and his life was crowded with melodrama. His name was Siebold.

Philipp Franz Balthasar von Siebold: A Lifelong Love for Japan

On August 8, 1823, the *Three Sisters*, flying the tricolor of The Netherlands and carrying the mission of Colonel der Steuler from Batavia, entered Nagasaki Bay.

As the sails were furled and the rudder shipped, a young German physician in the uniform of The Netherlands East Indies Army stood erect as a ramrod, gazing at the shores, seemingly unconcerned but inwardly entranced. Here was the moment that he had planned for months and lived for for years—the beginning of his life as a scientific explorer. He loved the green mountains that came down to the very shore, and even the foreboding lines of Deshima did not lessen his enthusiasm.

As the Hollanders moved from the ship to Deshima, each one was scrutinized and interrogated by the guards at the water gate. The young physician's heavy German accent was instantly detected and suddenly the guards refused to let him pass. Perhaps his long-held dreams were to be dashed. But der Steuler reacted with remarkable resourcefulness: "*Orandayama*, a Dutch mountaineer," he explained, and, fortunately for Japan and the Western world, the guards permitted Siebold to enter. Under these circumstances, Philipp Franz Balthasar von Siebold began a lifelong love affair with Japan; it was marked by great triumphs and deep tragedy.

Philipp Franz brought a rich intellectual heritage to his studies of Japan. He was one of the long line of scholarly Siebolds of the medical faculty at Würzburg University. The most eminent of his ancestors, his grandfather Karl Kaspar von Siebold (1736–1807), was, in the words of his colleagues, *Chirurgus inter Germanos princeps* (Leers). Karl Siebold brought Würzburg to the front ranks of medical schools in Germany, primarily through his lifelong dedication to the school and to the excellent teaching hospital, the Juliuspital. As a young man he had been sent to France, Holland, and Britain for medical studies by the bishop, Adam Friedrich von Sensheim, in return for which he had pledged to devote his life to advancing the medical faculty at Würzburg. Karl Siebold's main contributions were to surgery and obstetrics. He was a leader in raising surgery from the bloody practices of the barber-surgeons to the rank of an academic discipline. In obstetrics he developed the pelvic curve on the forceps. Obstetrics and midwifery held a special appeal for other members of the Siebold family. Among Karl Kaspar's pupils were his two nieces, who were the first German midwives to receive a postgraduate doctorate in obstetrics. One of them, Charlotte Heidenreich von Siebold, made the hurried trip from Germany to England with the pregnant Duchess of Kent, whose husband was determined that their baby should be born on British soil. Charlotte attended the duchess at the birth of her daughter on May 24, 1819, and eighteen years later the child became Queen Victoria.

The father of Philipp Franz, Johann Georg Christoph von Siebold (1767–98), was professor of physiology at Würzburg. Philipp was born on February 16, 1796, and his father died of tuberculosis just two years later. His mother, Maria Appolonia Josepha Lotz, was a responsible and forthright woman who raised her son with frequent advice from her brother, a priest at the Würzburg cathedral. In 1805 she moved her family to Heidingsfeld near Würzburg, and the following year they joined her brother's household.

The medical faculty at Würzburg was based in the Juliuspital, Germany's first teaching hospital. It was dedicated on March 12, 1576, by Bishop Julius Echter von Mespelbrunn for use as a military hospital in the religious wars that pitted Protestants against Roman Catholics. By direction of the prince-bishop, the citizens of his duchy were required to support the hospital by annual tithes from their harvests in grapes, agriculture, and timber. The hospital was the first in Germany to have an anatomical theater and a special neuropsychiatric facility, which were added in 1729.

Although severely damaged during the massive aerial assault on Würzburg in 1945, the hospital and anatomical theater have been restored. By the gate is a statue of Bishop Echter, and in one corner of the hospital is a highly popular *wein stube*. Its popularity is based in part on the superb *Frankenwein* that is made in the more than one hundred barrels that line the corridors of the basement of the hospital.

When in 1815 Philipp Siebold, at the age of nineteen, became the fifth member of his family to enroll in the Würzburg medical faculty, it was jokingly referred to as "Academica Sieboldiana." At this time he had the good fortune to move into the home of the professor of anatomy, Ignaz Döllinger, who was an important influence in encouraging Siebold's scholarly interests and thereby his career. Döllinger was a founder of the great line of anatomists and physiologists who led Germany to world-wide pre-eminence. He was distinguished for his studies on the maternal and fetal circulations. Another source of inspiration was the scholarly circle of Döllinger's scientific friends, led by the professor of botany at the University of Bonn, Christian Gottfried Daniel Nees von Esenbeck, which stimulated Philipp Franz to develop broad scientific interests. And, as an early sign of what was to become a lifelong dedication, tales of exploration were his favorite diversionary reading.

It was a most propitious era for the study of medicine in Germany for she was just beginning to take off in the remarkable leap that soon carried her to the zenith of medicine in the world. After his armies had been crushed by Napoleon in 1806, Frederick William III declared that "the State must make up in intellectual force what she has lost in physical" (Crawley, p. 118).

The University of Berlin was established in 1809 as the great national center of learning, but older institutions, such as Würzburg, Heidelberg, and Marburg, continued to thrive. Alexander von Humboldt preferred the intellectual spirit of Paris to that of the fatherland after his return from the Orinoco, but he was lured back to Berlin in 1827.

The *Geheimrat* ("secret counselor to the throne") professor was omnipotent and omniscient.* The most significant development in the German medical faculties was the establishment of research institutes with an emphasis on fundamental studies. This was in sharp contrast to the emphasis on the deadhouse and the dissecting room in the clinically oriented faculties of Britain and France. And, since the universities were the property of the individual states, or *Länder*, and not under national control, the faculties could vie quite openly for the best possible talent when chairs were vacant. Because of this mobility an able young scholar could be assured of an opportunity to ascend; he was not restricted to the line of succession at his own university. Soon it became almost obligatory for the medical faculties to turn outside when a professorial chair was vacated.

The curriculum in medical education was five and a half years in duration. The premedical courses included botany, chemistry, physics, comparative anatomy, and geology. The

---

* "Thou owest greater thanks to thy teachers than to thy father; he gave thee only bodily existence but they gave thee thy spiritual life" (cited in Magnus-Levy, p. 334). The quotation is from the Proverbs of the Fathers.

student then dissected a cadaver and, in some of the schools, studied topographical anatomy as well. Two semesters were devoted to physiology, and pathology was taught for an entire year. Materia medica included pharmacology, pharmacognosy, therapeusis, and toxicology. Clinical subjects were taught by lecture and demonstration in the amphitheater; the examination of patients was restricted to the polyclinic during the final year of study. It was customary for the graduate to spend two years in general practice to acquire clinical skills. There were infrequent but demanding examinations; each student was required to submit a set of statements for the final examination. Philipp Siebold's presentation on September 10, 1820, with thirty-five statements, was successful.

Siebold was active in the Corps Moenama, one of the many student societies which flourished in the German universities. * In contrast to the tradition that German students study in several universities, by his own choice he remained at Würzburg, largely because of his wish to be near his widowed mother. After ten semesters he completed his medical studies in 1820 with the academic rank of "excellent."

For two years Siebold "endured" general practice in the little town of Heidingsfeld. After one year the mayor described him as industrious and meticulous; his patients were quite satisfied. But he became increasingly restless and bored; he had the wanderlust that has affected so many Germans. He first turned to Philipp Jakob Cretzschmar at Frankfurt am Main in the hope that he would be sent to Brazil. When that request was unsuccessful, he turned, as did generations of his countrymen, toward seagoing Holland as the land of opportunity.

Fortunately, Franz Joseph Harbauer, a pupil of Siebold's father and an old friend of the family, was serving as director of hygiene of The Netherlands. There was need for an additional physician at The Hague, and Harbauer wished to discharge what he considered to be his educational debt to the memory of his former teacher. Through Harbauer, Siebold received the appointment, but court life in the drowsy capital held no opportunity for

* During World War II the society was called "Kameradschaft Philipp Franz von Siebold."

the life of a scientific explorer—which was his heart's desire. After a few months he requested a commission in the military forces for the East Indies. In a letter to a friend, Freiherr C. E. V. Moll, Siebold reaffirmed his devotion to natural history as the principal reason for his decision: "The love for the studies of natural history which from the cradle of my childhood went with me to the years of adolescence and under the leading of my forever beloved teacher, Döllinger, ripened with me to a man. This preference made me decide to take the major step to go to far away parts of the world" (translated from Körner, p. 808).

With characteristic German thoroughness, before sailing for the Orient, Siebold determined to spend a period acquainting himself with recent developments in natural history in Europe. For botany, he naturally turned to Bonn and the scientist whose company and wisdom he had enjoyed in the home of Döllinger, Nees von Esenbeck. Under his patronage Siebold was elected to membership in an esteemed scientific society, Kaiserliche Leopoldinische-Carolinische Akademie der Naturforscher, on June 26, 1822. On July 19 of the same year he returned to The Hague and was thrilled to learn that he had been appointed one of the four surgeon majors for the East Indies Army—and the youngest. Siebold had hoped to visit scientists in Brussels and the father of comparative zoology, Baron George Cuvier, in Paris, but since the sailing date of his ship was advanced, these visits were canceled.

On September 23, 1822, at the age of twenty-six, Philipp Franz von Siebold sailed from Rotterdam for Java. That he was enthusiastic and eager to reach Batavia we can be certain; that he hoped for an opportunity to visit Japan is quite probable. But neither he nor anyone else could have dreamed of the years of great achievement, love, happiness, and great despair that lay ahead. As a talisman he carried a strand of Döllinger's hair. When free from his duties as ship's surgeon, he collected marine biological specimens and studied Malay and Dutch.

After five months, on February 13, 1823, Siebold's ship dropped anchor at Batavia and he was assigned the duties of a regimental surgeon with the Fifth Artillery Regiment at Weltefreden. Restless in spirit, he found these duties boring and was delighted when

107

he was summoned to an appointment with the governor general, Baron van der Capellen, at his estate in Buitenzorg, near Batavia. In a letter to his Uncle Lotz, Siebold reported that the governor general had praised him as a new Kaempfer and Thunberg (*ibid.*, p. 812).

The baron was looking for a bright young physician to send to Japan as a scientific observer and collector, and the choice was a delicate and important one. The status of the Hollanders in Japan had declined when Raffles seized Batavia, and they were eager to regain their position. They believed that their status could be restored in part by a doctor who had the wide scientific interests and knowledge of Thunberg, who had been so popular in Japan. A second reason for the careful selection was the desire of the Dutch to bring up to date their information on all aspects of the culture of Japan. Russian, American, and English ships had intruded in Japanese waters and it was apparent that the Western nations were moving to force the opening of Japan to the West. The Dutch, still hoping for the role of favored nation when Japan was opened, felt that their chances would be enhanced if they continued to be the Western repository of knowledge on Japan.

The baron received an alert, intelligent young man who was poised and pleasant. Siebold's summer studies with Nees von Esenbeck now stood him in good stead. The range of his knowledge, his scientific interests, and above all, his burning desire for new intellectual conquests convinced van der Capellen that here was the man for Japan.

No physician had gone to Deshima with greater enthusiasm and opportunities for success than Siebold. His special scientific equipment included a galvanic apparatus, electrostatic generator, air pump, mariner's compass, and sextant. A lover of music, he included a pianoforte which he hoped would impress the Japanese, as well as the manuscripts of Kaempfer and Thunberg. As he sailed from Batavia with Captain Willem der Steuler, Siebold quoted Kaempfer, "*quid non mortalia pectora cogis/auri sacra fames*" ("to what lengths do you not drive the souls of men/infamous hunger of gold").*

* The quotation (cited in Wagner, p. 5211) is from Vergil's *Aeneid*, bk. 3, lines 56–57, as Aeneas is relating the story of Troy to Dido of Carthage.

Siebold's enthusiasm for Japan was heightened when the *Three Sisters* rescued the survivors of a Japanese ship that had sunk in a typhoon. In his diaries he recorded his respect for the courteous manner and the dignity of the Japanese survivors as they were brought aboard.

Siebold was almost ecstatic on his first landfall of Japan: "Calm winds and a clear sky unite to show the country in her most beautiful splendor. What inviting shores with their friendly homes! Those fertile hills, those majestic temples! How colorful do the green mountain summits appear in their volcanic formation! The richness of the evergreen oaks, cedars, and laurel trees" (translated from P. F. von Siebold, 1897, p. 42). It was love at first sight.

After their problem with Siebold's *Orandayama* on entering Deshima, Captain der Steuler and Siebold were delighted to be received by the departing *opperhoofd*, J. Cock Blomhoff, who had gathered a collection of Japanese art forms which impressed Siebold. He introduced Siebold to the Japanese physicians who were studying at Nagasaki; several were from as far away as Edo. With characteristic pride, Siebold noted that they as well as other learned doctors from distant communities had been drawn to Nagasaki by his reputation as the new Dutch doctor and natural scientist (*ibid.*, p. 120).

Siebold had been warned that at Deshima he would see a style of life which was of the previous century, characteristic of men withdrawn from the world, and he later wrote: "The formal politeness of these men among themselves and toward eminent Japanese, the old-fashioned clothes, embroidered velvet jackets and coats, hats with feathers, swords, and a Spanish cane with a huge golden knob—all this did not make the most favorable impression on us" (*ibid.*).

From the first day, Siebold threw himself into his new tasks with the inordinate zeal and meticulous scholarship that characterized his life: he studied the culture of the country, he taught, and he collected—especially natural history specimens which he classified. He recorded every impression in an exhaustive daily diary. For several hours each day he immersed his mind in the study of Japanese, and in books on Japanese literature and arts from which he was able to gain a background in the country's cultural traditions. His major contacts were with three of the interpreters, Narabayashi, Shige, and Nimura, who were his teachers on Japan. The eager Japanese students who came to Deshima every day were a source of inspiration for his lectures in medicine and natural history. Attracted by Siebold's excellence as a teacher, the number of students increased rapidly, and his room at Deshima soon became too small for his classes. Narabayashi, the scion of the historic family of interpreters, persuaded Nagasaki officials to permit Siebold to see patients and teach medicine and natural history at Narabayashi's home in Nagasaki City. Thus Siebold became the first foreigner to teach Western medicine systematically on the Japanese mainland.

An early disappointment for Siebold was related to smallpox vaccination. In his translation of *Shinsen Yōgaku Nempyō* by Ōtsuki Nyoden, Krieger reports that in 1795 a discussion of the importance of vaccination, *Shutō hitsujun*, was published by a practitioner, Ogata Shunsaku (Krieger, p. 107). When his town was ravaged by smallpox, Ogata, following the technique that he had learned in a Chinese medical text, powdered the scabs from patients and used the product for successful vaccinations. But, despite the use of vaccination in China, the Japanese did not adopt the procedure. Thus, when Siebold arrived, smallpox was widespread and he brought a small batch of immunizing lymph from Batavia to demonstrate the value of vaccination. On August 24, 1823, just sixteen days after his arrival at Deshima, he vaccinated two children, but the lymph had lost its potency and no vaccinia resulted. Siebold recognized the importance of vaccination and volunteered on several occasions to return to Batavia for active lymph, but the Japanese would not agree because they feared that the procedure would be harmful.

The commission from Baron van der Capellen was a source of great pride for Siebold and he worked day and night to fulfill it. Immediately after arrival he began to tap several sources for materials on every aspect of Japanese culture. His students, who paid no tuition, were aware of their teacher's interests and brought specimens of plant and animal life, and art works, as a sign of gratitude. His Excellency, the mayor of Nagasaki, gave Siebold permission to visit the city every second day and to collect specimens of botany and natural history in the city and in the suburbs. The interpreters were a third source of information and specimens. One of Siebold's patients, the director of the Royal Treasury in Nagasaki, even volunteered to go to the northern island of Japan, Ezo (now Hokkaido), to gather materials as a sign of his gratitude.

All plants or flowers that could be used as drugs or that were representative of Japanese horticulture were carefully transplanted to the garden at Deshima which had been developed by Kaempfer but which had deteriorated after Thunberg's return to Sweden. Siebold carefully laid out orderly plots for saplings, bushes, and plants. The specimens bore detailed labels and were divided equally between oriental and Western plants and flowers. Among the more important indigenous specimens were the sources of the drugs—important in the West—digitalis, belladonna, squill, and hyoscyamus.

For zoological specimens, in addition to the collections from his own expeditions and the gifts of students and interpreters, Siebold hired Japanese who were skillful hunters of wild game and birds. Many of the specimens were preserved and mounted while others, including foxes, monkeys, a wild boar, and a deer, were caged in an animal house next to the botanical garden at Deshima. On his expeditions to gather flora and fauna, Siebold was always accompanied by students led by Shige Dennoshin, who served in the three-way role of collector, guide, and interpreter. Two of the students, Gennosuke and Kumakichi, were taught to dry and press flowers and leaves and to mount animals and birds that had been brought in by the hunters. Siebold took special pride in the variety of specimens in the garden and in the animal house and pens at Deshima.

For specimens of marine life, Siebold joined the fish mongers at the seafood markets. No stone was left unturned in his ingenious dedication to executing the commission from van der Capellen, and each busy day and night brought fascinating new discoveries. So it was that just three months after his arrival in Nagasaki, the delighted young medical explorer wrote to his Uncle Adam: "I have arrived happily in Japan and spend the

111

most pleasant days of my life in restless activity in the fields of all of the natural and medical sciences. The most interesting land in the world for investigations has been granted to me. . . . I conduct lectures in the Dutch language on natural and medical science" (translated from Werner Siebold, 1943, pp. 36–37). He stated that he would send an annual paper on the medical problems and practices in Japan to Würzburg University.

Siebold's resourcefulness as a teacher and as a collector is best illustrated by his requirement that all students prepare dissertations in Dutch. Every topic assigned by Siebold related to some aspect of Japanese medicine, science, or culture: "On the Whales Produced in the Kyūshū Area"; "A Study on the Ancient History of Japan"; "A Method of Cultivating Tea Trees and Making Tea in Japan"; "A Short Catalogue and Record of All Illnesses Worthy of Attention Occurring in Japan"; "How to Make Salt"; "A Study of *Magatama* (A Method of Decoration of the Ancient People of Japan)"; "On the Cause of Measles and Smallpox in Children"; "The Acupuncture Method among the Chinese." With characteristic meticulousness, Siebold read every word, and all mistakes were corrected with a red pencil. In due course the dissertations were deposited in his rapidly expanding collections.

Siebold considered it one of his responsibilities to communicate his newly found knowledge to intellectual circles in Europe. In the first year he prepared three communications: on natural history in Japan; on Japanese obstetrics; and an epitome of the Japanese language illustrated with nine wood-block prints. These manuscripts were published first at Batavia and later in Germany and in Holland.

Siebold's diverse interests extended to comparative linguistics. He was tutored in Chinese as well as Japanese by the Nagasaki doctors. From shipwrecked Korean sailors at Nagasaki he learned of the syllabic alphabet used on the Korean peninsula. He promptly communicated this finding to the famed academy in Paris, but the linguistic experts in France did not accept his statements. Later, when he returned to Europe, he was able to exhibit materials that proved the validity of his earlier communication.

As Siebold's fame spread, physicians brought their problem patients to Nagasaki from distant communities for consultation;

the physicians joined the students in the lecture room at the completion of the consultation. Soon Narabayashi's house was too small and Siebold determined to try to obtain a larger building for his classes. Foreigners were forbidden to hold property in Japan, but Siebold's friend and student, Shige Dennoshin, acquired a lovely piece of property in the Narutaki section of Nagasaki which he turned over to Siebold. The house was seated on a spacious shelf of land on a steep hillside looking across a deep but narrow valley through which ran a pleasant stream. Siebold continued to live at Deshima, and in the one-mile walk to Narutaki he gathered fresh botanical and zoological specimens for demonstrations to his students.

Siebold was the first physician to systematically teach and demonstrate the practices of Western medicine and surgery in Japan. His diagnostic and therapeutic procedures were in sharp contrast to the reliance on pulse diagnosis, inspection of the tongue, and observation of the patient in *Kampō*. Whenever possible, he used patients for demonstrations of palpation and auscultation, the techniques for thoracic and abdominal paracentesis, and the use of belladonna in dilating the pupil. He received special acclaim for performing the first Western-style cataract surgery in Japan and for teaching the technique to his students. He introduced the use of the truss in the treatment of hernia, and surgical procedures for the repair of harelip, the removal of tumors of the breast, and hydrocele.

Siebold continued the family tradition of a special interest in obstetrics that had begun with his illustrious grandfather and continued with his aunts. He was the first to teach the use of the modern obstetrical forceps that his grandfather had pioneered in Europe, as well as operative procedures for difficult deliveries. He can be accurately described as the father of modern obstetrics in Japan. In materia medica he emphasized the use of aloes, antimony, cascara, calomel, digitalis, magnesia, and laudanum.

Siebold steadfastly refused to charge a fee for his medical services and thereby opened another source of materials for his collections; his patients expressed their gratitude with characteristic oriental gift-giving and literally showered him with scrolls, screens, books, pottery, and lacquerware.

After a year Siebold still was decidedly unimpressed with *Kampō*. It was his single disappointment in Japan.

The Japanese are unacquainted with the use of the practical metallic cauterizer and lance. There are a few exceptions, men who learned these skills from our surgeons. Nevertheless, with these very faults just mentioned, from their own genius they have adopted from the Chinese, who showed them the way, a twofold method of doctoring, so-called puncturing with needles and burning with moxa. Without these methods there would scarcely be any current practice of their medical art, for these bungling doctors, whose desire to eat is the motivating force of their talents and technique, know practically nothing about healing beyond what they have learned from our barbers, whose medical equipment is often minimal, or beyond what they have borrowed uncritically and untested from the writings of the Chinese, which few of them know well. As far as they are concerned, water is the universal solvent whether, as a remedy, it is derived from the animal, vegetable, or mineral kingdom, if you please. Indeed, I swear that so far I have discovered no illness among them which the doctor's lack of skill has not aggravated or worsened, and this ignorance has often caused the sick to die because of the very infrequent success of the treatment. This state of affairs pertains not only to the wealthy (for the poor die without help) but even to the very nobles of the realm, whose indelible hatred of Christianity causes them to choose a painful death rather then sensibly make use of our doctor's methods [translated from Archiv Mittelbiberach, 1968].

He complained that the Japanese doctors anointed even superficial lesions with so much medicine, in such varieties, and with so much bandage, that there was little opportunity for healing.

Later his attitude changed and he was astonished at the proficiency of some of the physicians in Japan. He was impressed with their zeal for Western knowledge; a new scientific publication in Dutch had become the most acceptable gift for a Japanese physician.

Literacy was as important in Japan in Siebold's period as it is today. All children were sent to primary school where they learned to read and write and were instructed in Japanese history. Those of higher rank were then instructed in arithmetic, astrology, etiquette, Confucian precepts—and when, where, and how to commit hara-kiri!

Letters from Thunberg, Döllinger, Schlegel, and Nees von Esenbeck lauded his studies and assured him of a triumphant return to the scientific community of Europe.

In 1825 Siebold's love for Japan took a different course when he met a beautiful and charming Japanese girl, Kusumoto Taki, at the home of one of his patients. Siebold was captivated. He learned that she was an eighteen-year-old geisha attached to a high-class house in the Maruyama quarter and that as a geisha she was called Sonogi ("fan"). Siebold asked Taki to join him on Deshima as his wife, but she was barred because only *yūjo* ("whores") were permitted to enter the island. However, she declared herself to be a *yūjo* instead of a geisha and in the winter of 1825 moved into Siebold's quarters on Deshima (Kure, 1896, p. 57). Itazawa, on the other hand, states that O-taki-san had always been a prostitute and was never a geisha (Itazawa, 1960, pp. 75–76). There were three classes of prostitutes in Nagasaki at this time, one for the Japanese, a second for the Chinese, and a third, *Oranda yuki* ("Dutch whore"), for the Hollanders. Sentiment of course favors the story that Taki was an honorable geisha who sacrificed her reputation by declaring herself a prostitute to join the man she loved. It is clear that Siebold held a deep affection for his wife, whom he called O-taki-san. For Siebold there was the added dividend that he could increase his fluency in Japanese, and in turn he taught O-taki-san Dutch. On May 10, 1827, at the little clinic on Deshima, Siebold delivered O-taki-san of a daughter, Ine, for whom he developed a deep and enduring devotion, which became mutual as the child grew older.

The need for accurate reproductions of his specimens as well as his desire to capture the colorful beauty of Japan made an artist an essential associate for Siebold. For the first year he relied on a talented young Japanese artist, Kawahara Keiga, whose father, also an artist, was a distinguished *Rangakusha* and had taught his son Western techniques in art. The wood-block prints prepared by Kawahara included illustrations of the wisteria, clematis, forsythia, hyacinth, acacia, peach, and pear. Illustrations of Japanese culture—the people, their customs, their habits, their diversions, as well as indigenous animals—were also represented in Kawahara's prints.

As early as November, 1823, three months after his arrival, Siebold asked the Dutch for an artist from Europe. In 1825 Karl Hubert de Villeneuve, an accomplished artist, came to Deshima to work with Siebold. Now Siebold had a team of artists, one skilled in Western techniques and one who could use the more traditional Japanese wood-block. Under Villeneuve's influence, Kawahara developed a greater facility for combining the Western use of perspective, shading, composition, expression, and detailed anatomy with the traditional Japanese art form. He became one of Japan's leading artists.

The Siebold study team was expanded further by the arrival of Heinrich Burger, a pharmacist and chemist from Batavia. The time of the arrival of Villeneuve and Burger was propitious, for Siebold was busy preparing for the *hofreis* to Edo.

Siebold on the Hofreis. For three years Siebold had looked forward to the day when he would begin the *hofreis* to Edo. He wished to inspect the great capital city and to exchange information with the physicians and scholars there who were far more advanced in *Rangaku* than his Japanese colleagues at Nagasaki. He hoped that he would be permitted to remain in Edo to extend his studies after the embassy had returned to Nagasaki. The one-thousand-kilometer journey by land and sea would afford exceptional opportunities to expand the fact-finding mission with which he had been charged at Batavia.

Shortly after his arrival at Deshima, Siebold had designed a red and blue frock coat edged with embroidery, after the style worn by the professors at Würzburg, which he proposed to wear on the *hofreis*.

The reduction of the *hofreis* to a quadrennial event in 1738 had been followed in 1790 by a limitation of the Dutch mission to just three persons, the *opperhoofd*, the doctor, and the secretary. It was essential that Villeneuve and Burger accompany Siebold to assist in his studies, and he was able to "smuggle" them into the retinue as his servants. A third "servant" was his leading student, Kō Ryōsai, who was fluent in Chinese and Dutch as well as in Japanese, and a fourth, Kawahara Keiga, completed the Siebold team.

116

They traversed the same route as their predecessors—across Kyūshū by land, from Shimonoseki on the beautiful Inland Sea to Murotsu near Himeji, and by land and sea to Edo with stops at Osaka, the great center of trade, and the lovely old capital seat of the mikado's court, Kyoto. The one-thousand-kilometer journey was divided into six hundred kilometers by land and four hundred kilometers by sea.

Siebold's voluminous diaries, observations, and collections from the *hofreis* indicate that he drove himself at a pace that was even more demanding than his grueling schedule at Nagasaki—and that he loved every minute of it. He was interested in everything; he was a perceptive observer, and his exhaustive records show that he was ever mindful of the need for information that would have military and strategic value. He worked seven days a week, eighteen hours a day, and he demanded a similar schedule from his assistants.

It is altogether possible that his almost flagrant disregard for the Japanese restrictions on the acquisition of information by members of the *hofreis* was a factor in the grave charges that were brought against him two years later.

Beyond medicine and natural history, geography and topography were his major interests. He carried a variety of instruments for his studies, including a barometer, altimeter, hygrometer, thermometer, microscope, sextant, and a chronometer; some of these he secreted in the lining of his hat. When the Japanese questioned him about his instruments and observations, he explained that they were necessary so that the clocks could be adjusted.

Siebold's diaries from the *hofreis* contain numerous examples of his wide range of interests and the exceedingly thorough manner in which he constantly applied himself to his studies. Infusions prepared from pulverized pearls were popular medicines. Siebold lists the scientific names of five mollusks that were sources of pearls; he learned that the pearls of one of the mollusks were used by Japanese and Chinese physicians for the treatment of abdominal cramps and diseases of the ears and eyes (P. F. von Siebold, 1897, p. 86).

117

The mystical practices of the Japanese to control the scourge of smallpox were striking to a European. At a village on the beautiful bay of Ōmura near Nagasaki, straw ropes plaited by *jammabosu* ("mountain priests") were hanging at the *genkan* ("entry") of the homes as a protection against an epidemic of smallpox which was raging. On the thresholds of afflicted individuals lay bamboo whisks to warn a possible visitor. Siebold noted that smallpox had been carried to Japan from Korea in the eighth century.

As the *hofreis* crossed Kyūshū, Siebold turned his attention to the volcanic spas that were as popular for medical therapy in Japan as in Germany. He recorded the color, taste, odor, and temperature of waters of each of the spas. As a further study he dropped eggs into the waters, and when he retrieved them in a few minutes they were boiled. The popularity of the springs in therapy ranged from patients with arthritis, smallpox, measles, and paralysis to those with chronic skin disease. It was encouraged by the fee which was so low as to be the equivalent of just one-fiftieth of a Dutch gulden. The reaction of the waters to eight chemical reagents, including lead acetate, ferrous sulfate, and barium hydrochloride, was tested by Burger. Although the waters seemed clear and pure, a sieve of human hair was used as a filter.

For his studies of marine biology Siebold caught seven species of fish and recorded their scientific names. His zoological studies included descriptions of the salamander and river otter. He recorded the methods used by the Japanese to trap wild ducks, geese, and cranes.

The utilization of native resources for Western naval expeditions was constantly a major consideration for Siebold. He visited a coal mine and noted that the products would be useful as fuel for ships. His observations were subsequently referred to in the official documents of the Perry expedition with its coal-burning vessels.

Siebold's success in Japan was due in no small part to his capacity for self-discipline. Every day was carefully scheduled. At times, therefore, he was irritated by the interruptions occasioned by the sudden appearance of his former students with patients for consultations or to present gifts and, at times, theses that he had assigned at Narutaki.

> At the crack of dawn, my pupils and other doctors of the neighborhood came with their sick and asked me for advice and assistance. The disorders were, as usual, chronic, neglected, and unhealable diseases, and the inconvenient consultations cost much time and patience. I did it all for my pupils' sakes whose good reputation would have suffered if their patients, to whom they had set me up as a source of comfort and whom they had often brought from the most distant places, had been sent away without advice or assistance. Thus, I often much against my will had to play the charlatan [translated from *ibid.*, p. 117].

This meeting with my most capable pupils was quite according to our agreement. They had received when they departed from their Dutch *meester* an impressive doctoral diploma with the understanding that they would write an inaugural dissertation which they would present to him on his trip to Edo. The title which was assigned to them was always on some unfamiliar subject that was worthy of study in the fields of geography, ethnography, or natural history in relationship to Japan and its neighboring lands and protectorates; for example, on that day:

—A description of the principalities of Nagato and Suwa.
—On the most common dyes and the colors of clothes.
—On whaling.
—Descriptions of the important diseases of Japan.
—A catalogue of the most common drugs [*ibid.*, p. 119].

The weeks in Edo surpassed Siebold's highest expectations. His fame had preceded him, and eighty miles south of Edo the *hofreis* was met by envoys sent to escort them through the feudatories to the capital city. Four decades had passed since Sugita, Maeno, and Ōtsuki had launched *Rangaku*, and now there were physicians and scientists in Edo who were familiar with Western science, who could speak Dutch, and who were able to ask intelligent questions and understand Siebold's answers.

Each day there were clinical demonstrations of the medical, surgical, and obstetrical procedures that he had introduced at

Nagasaki. His demonstrations on cataract surgery became exercises in comparative anatomy; he used a fish, then a swine that he had received as a gift, and finally, patients. There were many consultations for Japanese physicians. His physician-students included Katsuragawa Hoken, who now preferred the name Wilhelm Botanicus, which at his request he had been dubbed by a former *opperhoofd*, Hendrik Doeff. In gratitude for the consultations, demonstrations, and lectures, the Japanese physicians and their patients added many items to Siebold's collections. Others brought botanical and zoological specimens for him to identify, and frequently these too were added to his bulging chest of scientific treasures. Siebold in turn presented to each physician a list of medicines with indications for their usage which he had prepared with Kō Ryōsai.

On May 1, 1826, Siebold accompanied der Steuler and the secretary to the audience with the shogun, who was as usual screened from direct view. Der Steuler approached the invisible presence with the usual gifts and was required to lie prone on the mats as he deposited them. He, Siebold, and the secretary were then directed to make formal visits to the high officials of the *bakufu*, but: "Nowhere we found the dignitaries at home, everywhere we had to make our compliments to the secretaries, to sit exposed to all curious watchers, to smoke, to drink tea, eat candies, write down mottoes, and give away accessories over and over again. Finally, after fifteen hours, we came back with a headache and an upset stomach" (*ibid.*, p. 415).

On another visit to the court, while the *opperhoofd* discussed controversial aspects of the trade at Nagasaki with the *bakufu*, the court artists and scientists were constantly at Siebold's side. They showed him many pieces of art and escorted him to the libraries of Edo to view imperial treasures. The court botanist presented a *kakemono* which depicted specimens of marine life from the seas of Japan and China. Another representative of the court who paid him homage was the official acupuncturist, who placed in his hands a lengthy treatise on the techniques of both acupuncture and moxibustion. The geographer to the *bakufu*, Mogami Tokunai, had made an expedition to Sakhalin and gave Siebold an invaluable map proving that the territory was an island and not a peninsula. According to Siebold the reason for such a valuable gift was "so that it would not be lost for science" (*ibid.*). Siebold's interest in comparative linguistics naturally led him to a lengthy discourse with Mogami on the language of the Ainu, on which he subsequently published a treatise.

The most rewarding yet ultimately destructive relationship that Siebold established on the *hofreis* was with the court astronomer, Takahashi Sakuzaemon, also known as Kageyasu. Hendrik Doeff had dubbed him Globius. Siebold was constantly on the lookout for materials of military significance. Takahashi was the keeper of the Great Map of the Japanese coastlines, which was based on careful surveys and was therefore of surpassing strategic importance. The map was closely guarded, available to only a few Japanese, and under no circumstances was to be shown to a foreigner. We do not know if Siebold was aware of the existence of the map before he met Takahashi, but with Siebold's propensity for ferreting out information it is quite possible that he did. To win his favor and encourage an exchange of information, Siebold presented Takahashi with a map of Russia and a copy of a book by the famed Russian admiral, A. J. von Krusenstern (Krusenstern, 1810–12 and 1814). In return Takahashi brought the imperial secret map of Inō Tadataka for Siebold to study at a dinner which Siebold gave for the physicians and scientists of the court. Takahashi agreed to have a copy of the map prepared and to send it to Siebold at Nagasaki, which he did through an interpreter, Yoshio Chūjirō.

Since the Great Map was the major factor in Siebold's subsequent banishment from Japan, a note on its significance is relevant. Inō Tadataka, also known as Chūkei (1745–1818), a former brewer, between 1800 and 1816 carried out the first detailed survey of the coastlines of Japan from Ezo (Hokkaido) in the north to the southwestern end of Kyūshū, including the island of Shikoku. Several maps of Japan had been prepared previously, one dating back to the middle of the seventeenth century:

> Although they were fairly well compiled from the data presented by each *daimyō* in their accuracy and detail they were far behind Inō's map which was based on actual survey. . . . The coastline and place-names along the surveyed roads are

in detail and accurate, but hills and mountains are mostly depicted in profile, and in middle- and small-scale maps, with abundance of azimuth lines from various points along the roads to the prominent peaks. Hills and mountains are shown in dark green, rivers are in blue, the configuration of the coast is bordered by light blue, azimuth lines in red, *kanji* (Chinese characters) of place names are well written, and all are in balance and in harmony and the maps give even an impression of a work of art, which suggests that Inō had a number of assistants who were skilled in drawing beautiful maps [Hoyanagi, p. 150].

Using instruments which were solely of his own design, Inō made nine expeditions ranging in distance from 1,500 to 5,500 kilometers. He died before the map was completed, and the drawings were prepared by a group of students under the supervision of Takahashi Sakuzaemon, whose father, Takahashi Yoshitoki, had been a teacher and colleague of Inō. The last of the copies based on Inō's surveys was presented to the *bakufu* in 1821, just five years before they were shown to Siebold. The map was on three scales: there were more than 200 sheets for the large scale, 8 sheets for the middle scale, and 3 sheets for the small scale. Fortunately Inō made several copies of each map so that, despite fire and earthquake, copies are available today at the Inō Museum in Sawara City, Chiba Prefecture, and a copy of the small-scale map is preserved at the National Maritime Museum in Greenwich, England.

Before the *hofreis* Siebold had hoped that he would be allowed to remain in Edo after his associates returned to Nagasaki, and the wealth of information that flowed to him during it only heightened his ambitions. His Japanese colleagues, who were eager for him to remain, were optimistic about his chances, but der Steuler's disagreement with the *bakufu* over the Nagasaki trade became so pronounced that on May 18, 1826, the Hollanders were ordered to return immediately to Nagasaki. Henceforth relations between Siebold and der Steuler deteriorated steadily, in part because of the *opperhoofd*'s jealousy and petulance, and in part because of Siebold's aggressiveness and haughtiness.

On the return trip to Nagasaki they enjoyed Kabuki plays at the Kadoza theater in Dotonbori, Osaka. One of the plays was

Mōtei no kyoku ("The Song of the Blind Emperor"), from Imo-seyama Onna Teikin. It was a *jōruri*, or ballad drama, written in 1771 by Chikamatsu Hanji, Chikamatsu Tonen, Matsuda Baku, and Sakai Zenpei. The play was the basis for an interesting relationship in the twilight of Siebold's career. According to one of his biographers: "He was deeply moved by the plot and wrote in his diary, *Edo Sampu Nikki*, on June 12, 1826, a detailed description of the performance and of the contents of the play" (translated from Kure, 1926, p. 520).

Briefly, the story tells of an emperor, Tenchi, who is driven from the throne and stripped of his imperial insignia because of sudden blindness. An impoverished hunter near Nara hides the refugee-emperor in his hut and tries to restore his vision by giving him blood stolen from the sacred deer at Nara. The hunter is sentenced to execution for violating the deer, but his sons in filial piety volunteer to take his place on the block. However, before the execution, courtiers from the imperial palace enter the hut bearing the lost imperial crests, the emperor's vision is instantly restored, and the hunter and his family are pardoned.

Despite the mounting antagonism with der Steuler, Siebold was able to collect many specimens and to continue his observations on the return trip. Several Edo doctors accompanied him as volunteers for a major part of the journey and listed for Siebold the Japanese and Chinese names of the more than one thousand botanical specimens that he had accumulated. On July 7, 1826, Siebold, probably the happiest man in Japan, walked through the gates of Deshima. The journey had taken five months, and his achievements had exceeded his wildest dreams.

The problems raised by the hostility of der Steuler seemed to be resolved when the *opperhoofd* was recalled to Batavia at the insistence of the *bakufu*. However, der Steuler continued his bitter complaints to the officials at headquarters and several of der Steuler's friends who remained at Deshima were openly antagonistic to Siebold.

Confinement and Expulsion from Japan. When he returned to Nagasaki, Siebold spent most of the day and night in identifying and preserving the hundreds of scientific, cultural, and artistic specimens that he had gathered on the *hofreis*, but he continued

123

to teach medicine, natural history, and Dutch. He wrote to Nees von Esenbeck that his Japanese students were especially valuable in assisting him in his studies on botany and linguistics, and he enclosed a manuscript in which he described two hundred and fifty plants. In a letter to his mother on December 12, 1827, Siebold expressed great satisfaction in his accomplishments as the end of his term approached (Körner, p. 842).

Siebold planned to return to Europe in the fall of 1828 to establish his role as the Western authority on Japan. In due course he would return to Japan to continue his studies and to renew his happy life as a Japanese husband and father. He looked forward to the accolades of the departing hero and a triumphal return to Europe. But tragedy struck. He was arrested by the Japanese for having a copy of the imperial map, confined to Deshima, and, after a year, expelled—never to return. It was a tragic end to six glorious years. The circumstances were partly of his own making, as well as evidence of the last-ditch stand of Japanese reactionaries against foreign influence.

As the years had passed at Deshima, Siebold's status with the *Rangakusha* had risen to heights reserved for a *daimyō*. He became increasingly aggressive and self-assured and completely ignored the fact that it was still necessary for a foreigner, even Siebold, to be circumspect in gathering information. He became enchanted with a self-portrait that he saw in his dreams—Europe's leading authority on Japan; counselor to emperors and kings; the leader in opening Japan to the West. The adulation of the *Rangakusha* elevated his already soaring self-esteem.

In his path stood the Neo-Confucianists, now with their backs to the wall, desperate to destroy *Rangaku* and to terminate any efforts at expanded Western contacts. They saw the imperious Siebold, who they knew was a German masquerading as a Hollander, as a prime target and they were determined to bring him down. The role of his Dutch enemies at Deshima is unclear, but there were certainly members of the staff, including friends of der Steuler, who would not protect Siebold or who might even have informed on him for possessing contraband.

The story of Siebold's downfall is filled with sheer melodrama —informers, the purloined map, buried secrets, a typhoon-wrecked ship, and friends urging *seppuku*. Siebold received orders from Batavia to sail for Java on the *Cornelius Houtteman*, an East Indiaman, in the fall of 1828. On September 18, 1828, the *Houtteman*, with eighty crates containing the final shipment of Siebold's collections aboard, foundered in a typhoon at Inasa near Nagasaki. When the hulk was inspected Siebold's collections were discovered, including forbidden maps and a *haori* bearing the shogun's crest. To complete the catastrophe the Nagasaki authorities, representing the *bakufu*, were informed that Siebold had a copy of the Great Map of Inō Tadataka and that it had been given to him by the court astronomer, Takahashi Sakuzaemon. Although sworn to secrecy by officials who had crossexamined him, one of Siebold's students came to warn him of his impending arrest. With the hope that he might be able to save Takahashi, who had been arrested with thirty-two of Siebold's students, Siebold stayed at his desk all night to make a copy of the Great Map so that he could surrender the copy from Takahashi in the morning. It is probably for this reason, a hurried all-night transcription under great tension, that the map of Japan which Siebold circulated in Europe has been described by Hoyanagi as a "map rather inaccurately compiled by Siebold" (p. 158).

Siebold was able to bury materials at Deshima and at Narutaki; small items were secreted in the animal cages before his arrest and confinement at Deshima. The *opperhoofd* Meylan dared not intervene with the xenophobic Japanese at a time when flagging Dutch fortunes were just beginning to rise—in no small part because of Siebold's outstanding work. Since Meylan remained aloof Siebold began to suspect that the Dutch had joined the intrigue against him. The situation became so desperate that Siebold's friends smuggled in the short, straight sword to suggest that he should follow the samurai code and commit *seppuku*. His morale was bolstered by O-taki-san, who was constantly at his side.

The arrest in no way diminished Siebold's determination to be a collector. He raised a female goat so that his students could conceal botanical specimens in the fodder. When the next ship arrived from Batavia they began to smuggle aboard specimens and other materials from Narutaki as well as from Deshima. They were so successful that Siebold left Japan with most of the collection that he would have carried as a free man.

Siebold insisted that his studies had no relation to espionage, and he could not be persuaded to release the names of the Japanese who had passed materials to him. After a year the king of Bavaria, at the urging of Siebold's mother, requested William I to intercede. In view of his contributions as a doctor and teacher, Siebold was pardoned and exiled in October, 1829. He sailed from Nagasaki on January 2, 1830, six years and three months after the day when he had stood enraptured by his first sight of Japan.

It was a deadly blow to Siebold's pride; he could never return to his beloved Japan. His dreams of playing the major role at Edo when the empire was opened to the West were dashed. His personal loss was heightened by his devotion to his little daughter, Ine, just two years old. As he had carried Döllinger's hair with him to Japan, he carried locks of Ine's and O-taki-san's hair to Europe, and he commissioned a Japanese artist to prepare their portraits to be sent to him. He entrusted the care of his wife and daughter to Kō Ryōsai, to whom he gave his medical and surgical instruments.

Siebold's Followers. Siebold bequeathed to Japan a talented band of young scholars in his former students. One of them, Takano Chōei (1804–50), pursued a career in many respects as interesting, as scholarly, as varied, and as turbulent as that of Siebold. He has been described as "probably the most accomplished Dutch scholar of his day in Japan" (Sansom, 1962, p. 260). The son of a medical family at Mizusawa, Iwate Ken, near Sendai in northeast Japan, Takano began the study of medicine in Edo at the age of sixteen and supported himself by working as a masseur. After five years of study he determined to learn Dutch and enrolled with Siebold at Narutaki. When he had completed his studies he entered the service of the *daimyō* of Hirado Island, the seat of the Dutch and British factories when they first came to Japan. He dedicated himself to a life of scholarship in translating and writing books that he hoped would bring benefit to his country and credit to his parents. But at this rewarding stage in Takano's career Siebold was arrested and Takano, fearing for his own safety because of his many translations, fled to Satsuma and hid. After the turbulence precipitated by the Siebold affair had waned, Takano made his way stealthily to Hiroshima where he continued to hide. Here he was found by Ono Ryōsaku, a former student of his stepfather, who insisted, against Takano's protests, that he return to his native village to rejoin his parents. Takano refused to go farther north than Edo; to return to his birthplace would mean the abandonment of his idealistic plans for service to his country. He expressed this attitude to Ryōsaku: "It is an ultimate goal of filial piety to hand one's name down to posterity by making success" (translated from Fukushima, p. 156). And he composed a poem to indicate his dreams for the future: "Science prevails in western countries/and my eyes are looking at five continents/ I expect that, after my accomplishments/the world will appreciate their benefits" (*ibid.*). To make his dedication to the study of Western learning complete, Takano severed his connections with the Date clan by feigning illness and became a scholarly *rōnin.*

Fortunately for Takano Chōei, his decision to remain in the shogun's city coincided with a resurgence of interest in *Rangaku* to a point where a physician to the shogun, Matsumoto Ryōsuke, quite openly advocated the adoption of Western medicine. Soon Takano had a wide circle of friends in Edo, principally among men who were Dutch scholars and who publicly advocated the opening of the country. This environment was ideal and Takano busied himself with writings and translations. To medicine his most important contribution was *Igen sūyō*, published in 1836; it was the first modern physiology text written in Japan. For sources, Takano used primarily a Dutch translation of a German text by Johann Friedrich Blumenbach. The range of his writings was remarkable: on public health, *Control of Communicable Diseases*; on clinical medicine, *Principles of Syphilis* and *Principles of Obstetrics*. During a severe famine, he published *Two Principles in Preventing Devastation*. Among his non-medical publications were *Outline of Dutch History* and *Collection of Curiosities*. But one publication, *Yume Monogatari* [A tale of a dream], was a fatal mistake. In it Takano described the progressive state of affairs and the interest-

127

ing customs in other countries, using England as his primary example. His sin was that he advocated in this book the opening of Japanese ports to the Western powers. This was directly in opposition to *bakufu* policy and immediately drew him to the attention of the police. He compounded his problems by overindulging in sake, which was one of his favorite pastimes, and shouting on the streets about the stupidity of the shogunate. This brought him under constant scrutiny of the police, who were only awaiting an opportunity to arrest him. Rather than have the *bakufu* charge his former master, Lord Date, with treason, Takano turned himself in to the police and was promptly imprisoned. After five years in jail, during which he continued to write articles, his prison was threatened by one of the conflagrations that periodically ravaged large parts of Edo. All prisoners were freed with the commitment that they would voluntarily return to prison in three days. Takano visited his mother and, instead of returning to the prison in Edo, hid himself again. Fortunately, the descendant and successor to his former *daimyō* was willing to hide him, and Takano was reported dead. But after one year he determined to return at all costs to Edo; for disguise, he burned his face with gunpowder and changed his name. But his drive and ability caught up with him. With two associates he translated a book on military strategy from Dutch into Japanese and the quality of the translation was so good that Takano's existence was promptly recognized; it could be attributed only to Takano Chōei. On October 30, 1850, he was seized by a band of police at Hyakunin-chō, Aoyama, in Edo. After slaying one of the policemen, he endeavored to commit *seppuku* but missed the vital spot and ignominiously bled to death in the mud.

Almost fifty years later, in September, 1898, Takano's achievements were recognized by the court and he was honored with the award fourth court rank, senior grade. At that time a monument was erected at Zenkōji Temple, near the place where he died, with an epigraph that reads in part: "Alas! It was this book on tactics. Because of it you lost your life. Because of it the government now confers posthumous honors on you . . . [for] the world has entirely changed, and the new era has come today. This country certainly owes the present prosperity to those forerunners who made contributions at the sacrifice of themselves. Criminals in old days are now considered as loyal citizens. I simply regret it with a deep sigh. . . . Kaishū Katsu Yasuyoshi." At 6–5, *chōme*, Minami-Aoyama, a plaque marks the place where Takano hid on the night of his death: "This is the historic spot where Takano Chōei hid himself on the night of October 30, 1850 (the third year of Kaei). This was the detached house of Iseya, a pawnshop owned in olden times by a shogun's retainer at Hyakunin-chō, Aoyama. Here he concealed himself and breathed his last."

Other students of Siebold were less heroic than Takano Chōei but played important roles in the advance of Western medicine in Japan. Itō Genboku, Totsuka Seikai, and Takeuchi Gendō were the first Western-trained physicians appointed as court physicians to the shogun. These appointments were made in 1858 as futile efforts to save the life of the shogun, Tokugawa Iesada, who was dying of beriberi.

Kō Ryōsai opened a practice in ophthalmology in Osaka, where he also established in 1836 a school, Chōzendo, to teach Western medicine. He soon became Japan's leading eye surgeon, but several of his papers on ophthalmology were banned from publication because they contained information that he had gathered from Siebold. The Japanese officials stated: "Although these writings seem to be of use to the public, they contain on several occasions the name of von Siebold, a man persecuted by us. Ryōsai has all the reasons to feel respect and gratitude for his former teacher; but since von Siebold is guilty of having violated the laws of the country, his name must disappear from these books before the publication can be granted" (translated from Kleiweg de Zwaan, p. 517). When all references to Siebold had been deleted, the books were published; the most important was *Jigan Shōsetsu* [Detailed explanation of the ear and eye].

Siebold's students made major contributions to the development of other fields of Western surgery, as well as to ophthalmology, in Japan. The three leaders were Totsuka Seikai, Homma Genchō, and Ninomiya Keisaku. Nor were Siebold's leading students restricted to medicine. Kozeki Sanei translated Western astronomy texts for the court at Edo and later joined a group,

Shoshikai, with Takano Chōei, which aspired to serve as an advisory council on political and economic problems to the feudal lords. Iwasaki Kanyen was a distinguished botanist.

Siebold in Exile. The excellence of his students and his massive collections were of little consolation to Siebold as his ship sailed down Nagasaki Bay, carrying him to a lifelong expulsion from Japan. When they reached Batavia, Siebold immediately went to the gardens at Buitenzorg to identify and study plants that he had shipped from Nagasaki. Many were in bloom; his most important botanical contribution had been the Japanese tea plant, which had already become the foundation of a flourishing tea culture in the Indies.

The contraband that poured from the decks and holds of Siebold's ship at Batavia was a remarkable testimonial to his success in Japan. It revealed a harvest of more than 5,000 zoological specimens, including 900 birds, 750 fish, 200 mammals, and 170 reptiles. There were an equal number of botanical specimens, the most valuable of which he acclimatized with his other plants in the gardens at Buitenzorg in anticipation of the long voyage to Europe. He had fulfilled beyond all expectations the mission assigned by Baron van der Capellen at Buitenzorg more than six years earlier.

Before the departure from Batavia, Siebold hired a Chinese, Tschang, to accompany him to Holland and serve as a linguistic assistant in the extensive publications on Japan which he projected.

Exhausted in mind and body, Siebold welcomed the long sea voyage to Rotterdam. Yet he was absorbed in maintaining at all costs the living specimens in his botanical collection: he inspected each of the specimens daily, and plants that appeared to be losing their viability were placed on the masts with the hope that the sea breezes would restore them.

When Siebold landed in Holland in July, 1830, the country was in revolt; the southern provinces had declared their independence from The Hague and had established themselves as Belgium. Because this separation involved the great seaport of Antwerp, it was a serious financial as well as prestigious blow, not only to the Dutch, but also to Siebold, who had planned to sell his collection to King William I. Some of Siebold's prized specimens had been planted in the gardens of Ghent, but they were regained.

Siebold's spirits were revived by the recognition granted him the following spring. On April 11, 1831, the king awarded him the Cross of the Dutch Lion, and on the thirtieth of that month Siebold was promoted to the special rank of commander of medical welfare of The Netherlands East Indies Army and adviser on Japanese affairs. He was decorated by the king of his native Bavaria and received an honorary doctorate in philosophy at Würzburg. His personal happiness was increased by letters in broken Dutch from O-taki-san, who told of his cherished Ine.

The inability of the financially depleted court at The Hague to purchase his collection did not deter Siebold, his old energy restored, from undertaking the demanding tasks of classifying and arranging his Japanese collections and preparing manuscripts from the mass of information he had gathered in Japan. He decided to settle in Leiden, primarily because of the strong oriental programs at the university, and purchased a house at 19 Rapenburg, just a few blocks from the medical faculty.

Siebold was a complete individualist and guarded the independence that let him live the life of an intellectual explorer. In a letter to his mother on September 21, 1830, he stated that he had a full program for the next ten years and must remain free (Körner, p. 853). His sole concern was for Japan; he was dedicated to documenting his studies and to keeping an eye on the welfare of his adopted fatherland. Therefore, he had no interest in the life of a professor. His attitude could not have been expressed more directly than when he described the change that would have occurred if he had shifted from his life in Japan to a European professorship as a shift from "the pace of a horse to the pace of an ass." He was far too much of an individualist to accept an academic career— even with the freedom of the highly autonomous professor in a European university.

The lovely flowers and plants that Siebold had nurtured so carefully on the long voyage from Batavia to Holland were his closest link to his beloved Japan. To see their offspring as permanent additions to European gardens was his major objective.

131

Siebold decided that this would be best accomplished by exhibiting them in the setting of a classical Japanese garden. He purchased a large plot of land at Lagan Rijndik in the village Leiderdorp near Leiden and designed a garden to follow the beautiful settings that he had enjoyed at Nagasaki, Kyoto, and Edo. Here he planted Japanese specimens of the magnolia, clematis, glycine, peony, and hydrangea, as well as the cherry, peach, oak, maple, pine, and the classical bamboo. To assure the success of their cultivation, he constructed a hothouse which he referred to as his *Jardin d'Acclimatation*. The garden at Leiderdorp was the first major display in Europe of oriental trees, plants, and flowers growing in a garden of oriental design. Quite naturally Siebold was delighted when it soon became a "required course" for foreign dignitaries from The Hague. The first distinguished foreign visitor represented a country that played a crucial role in Siebold's future. He was the czarevitch, who later became Alexander II of Russia. To further his goal of introducing Japanese botany to Europe, Siebold donated seeds and shoots to the major botanical institutes of the European countries.

In the summer of 1834 Siebold embarked on a tour of selected European capitals. The major reason was to obtain commitments and if possible advance payments for the purchase of copies of his publications on Japan; the program at Leiden had depleted his purse. He also wished to establish his role in foreign intellectual circles as the Western expert on Japan and to stimulate interest in that country.

The grand tour exceeded Siebold's highest expectations: he was received by nobility; he was decorated; and, to his greatest satisfaction, he was honored in Russia. His first stop was in St. Petersburg where he arrived at the same time as did the members of a Russian caravan that had been trading with the Chinese on the Manchurian border. From them he gathered information on the state of affairs in Japan. He also met the famous circumnavigator, Admiral A. J. von Krusenstern, whose book had been a factor in Siebold's tragedy in Japan. In one of their discussions of the Far East, Siebold showed Krusenstern his maps of Japan, China, and Russia and Siebold noted in his diary that he was the first person to inform Krusenstern that Sakhalin was an island and not a peninsula.

Delighted with his reception and with the Russians, Siebold remained in Moscow for an entire month. The czar offered him an appointment as adviser to the court which Siebold declined; his first commitment was to complete his studies and writing. He was decorated by the czar with the order Vladimir, class IV, and the regent also ordered ten copies of *Nippon*. The Kaiserliche Gesellschaft der Naturforscher awarded Siebold an honorary diploma and when he went to Berlin he was given an audience with the prince and was decorated. But the most important event on his calendar in Berlin was the opportunity to establish a lasting acquaintance with the famed explorer of the Orinoco and the Andes, Baron Alexander von Humboldt. When Siebold reached Munich, the capital of his native Bavaria, he proposed to King Ludwig I the establishment of an ethnographic museum and enlisted the services of Joseph Gerhard Zuccarini, a botanist, to work with him at Leiden. In Vienna he was moved deeply when the emperor recalled the contributions of Siebold's father and grandfather in medicine, and Siebold was flattered by the enthusiasm that Prince Metternich expressed for his programs.

The discussions of an ethnographic museum in Munich only strengthened Siebold's resolve to see a similar project undertaken in Leiden to house his collections. He believed that in such a setting they might well stimulate an enthusiasm for Japan that would result in direct intercourse between Europe and the Island Empire. In a thoughtful and provocative memorandum Siebold set forth his ideas for "a scientificially arranged exhibit of materials from many countries—primarily from outside Europe —to give a clear mental picture of the state of their arts and sciences, economy, crafts and skills in art, and their trade." He pointed out that since the economy of The Netherlands relied on trade and commerce, such a museum would be useful for all men, from ambassadors to sailors, preparing for overseas service. His respect for Japanese culture is clearly evident in the memorandum: "We should recognize that excellent qualities and abilities in the non-European—even art and science—are not strange to even the people most remote to us. . . ."* Finally, he recom-

---

* The memorandum is in the archives of the National Ethnographic Museum in Leiden.

mended that, because of its completeness, the Japanese collection should be the first deposition.

In 1837, with some of the financial strain of the Belgian separation eased, the Dutch government puchased the collection and installed Siebold as the curator of the National Ethnographic Museum at Leiden, the first such museum in Europe.

The variety and number of Japanese specimens that Siebold deposited at the museum in Leiden is another testimonial to the scope of his interests and the extent of his collections: *Katalogus der Verzameling van den Heere Von Siebold* lists a total of 1,468 volumes of books, atlases, and charts at the museum: depictions of the Japanese way of life; dictionaries; descriptions of Nagasaki, Tokyo, Osaka, and Kyoto; histories; religious books and tracts; vital statistics; and a wide variety of art forms.

To the visitor in 1969, the collection is still impressive; it includes more than twenty meticulous scale models of Japanese homes, shops, and other public buildings. Many stand more than two feet high, with interiors and furniture carefully duplicated; inspection of the buildings is facilitated by removable roofs and floors. There are a number of models of the unique Japanese ships with no stern area that were the only seagoing vessels permitted by the Tokugawa *bakufu*. The buildings and ships were obviously prepared by highly skilled Japanese craftsmen at what must have been significant cost to Siebold.

There is a complete model of Deshima with about forty buildings—warehouses, offices, residences—and the famed botanical garden is shown adjoining the home of the factory doctor and his clinic. More than one hundred dolls depict a procession of samurai led by their *daimyō*, while other dolls represent ceremonial figures. There is a large collection of the puppets that form such an important part of the Japanese Noh theater. As a memento of Japanese physicians, there are several miniatures of the long, straight steel sword of the samurai, but they are only eighteen inches long and are made of wood instead of steel. They are the facsimile or "surrogate" swords that physicians were permitted to wear as a sign of their special rank.

Visited by nobility from The Hague, honored in the courts of Europe, Siebold was shunned by the people of Leiden. They considered him an eccentric, and he apparently took pleasure in filling that role. He delighted in walking the streets of the sedate university town in traditional Japanese costume. In the winter he frequently dressed for public display in a knee-length lined cloak, or *haori*, and a divided skirt (*hakama*); in the summer he wore a loose-fitting kimono.

The professors and burghers of Leiden saw a strange pair when the tall, erect, bearded Siebold, in his Japanese costume, was accompanied by his short Chinese assistant, Tschang, dressed in mandarin style, with a long queue. And the sight of a European with an Oriental walking beside him as a colleague rather than following at an appropriate distance, as was the custom in The Netherlands as well as in Java, was particularly galling to the Dutchmen.

At his home at Leiderdorp, Siebold led a combined Japanese-European style of life which added to his reputation as an eccentric. He frequently slept on *tatami* mats in the manner of Japanese, held conversations with visitors seated on the floor mats, and removed his shoes before entering the house.

Siebold had a penchant for unusual people. The gate was guarded by a strange old man who, with a sickle that he held as a weapon, resembled Father Time. He was interested in the problems of a man who did nothing but fish—night and day. He joined a band of wandering Jews as they traversed Holland. It was no wonder that the burghers of Leiden, in contrast to the nobility of The Hague, came to Leiderdorp to catch a glimpse of this strange explorer and his retinue rather than to view his botanical gardens.

Siebold recruited an effective team of assistants in addition to Zuccarini, the Munich botanist, for his studies and publications. For linguistics he was joined by Johann Joseph Hoffman, a fellow native of Würzburg whom Siebold met when Hoffman was touring Holland with a singing group. For zoology he enlisted the aid of another German, H. Schlegel, from Saxony; and for ethnographic studies he secured C. J. Temminck, the curator of the Rijksmuseum. But the domineering and *geheimrat* manner of Siebold made the association finally unbearable for his assistants —one worked for Siebold but never with him! Eventually his

135

assistants left in despair, but fortunately, because of the fascination of studying completely new fields, they tolerated Siebold long enough to see the three major works to fruition. One of these, which appeared appropriately with Siebold as the sole author, was *Nippon*. It is a truly massive documentation of Siebold's diaries from his six years in Japan; the most important section is his detailed description of the *hofreis* to Edo. *Nippon* has never gained the stature as a reference source on Tokugawa Japan that was achieved by Kaempfer's great book, nor is it as interesting to read as Thunberg's *Travels*. *Nippon* served as the primary source for a description of life in Japan edited by Busk and published in 1841. It gained popularity at the time of the opening of Japan to the West.

The second publication of the trilogy was the most pioneering, *Fauna Japonica;* it was the first comprehensive description of the fauna of the Far East to be published in the West. The four volumes describe in detail the birds, mammals, fish, and shellfish of Japan with excellent illustrations.

The third book was *Flora Japonica*, with J. G. Zuccarini as the co-author. It included descriptions of a number of Japanese plants, such as the hydrangea and the peony, which were first cultivated in Europe from Siebold's acquisitions in Japan.

In the winter of 1839–40, Siebold visited Würzburg where he met the von Gagern family. Hans von Gagern was impressed with Siebold's deep feeling for Japan: "The most interesting person whom I have met is Siebold. . . . in his heart he is still completely Japanese and would return there immediately" (translated from Körner, p. 879). Siebold and Hans von Gagern established a close friendship and Siebold visited the family in Würzburg on several occasions. On July 10, 1845, in Berlin, at the age of fifty, Siebold married Hans's twenty-five-year-old sister, Helena Caroline Frein von Gagern. Siebold and his bride established themselves in a new home at Leiderdorp which he, not surprisingly, named "Nippon." In a year the first of five children, a son, Alexander, was born. Hans von Gagern, fascinated by Siebold's stories of Japan, came to Leiden in the autumn of 1846 to study Siebold's collections in anticipation of accompanying him when he returned to Japan. He assisted Siebold in the preparation of *Nippon* and noted in his diary that Siebold's facility in German had suffered because of his six years in Japan.

In 1847 Frau Siebold contracted malaria and Siebold reluctantly decided to move to the Rhineland. He chose as his home an old nunnery, St. Martin, near Boppard, about ten miles south of Koblenz, but returned to "Nippon" in Leiden for the summer months.

Siebold maintained continuing contact with The Hague through the lifetime citizenship as a "Jonkheer" of The Netherlands which he had been awarded in 1842. The future of the Dutch in Japan was a major concern of the court at The Hague, and they relied on Siebold as an adviser on oriental relations. In January, 1848, he was promoted to the rank of colonel in The Netherlands army and placed on official leave so that he could continue to live abroad.

During these years Siebold had no direct line of communication with Japan; he could not enjoy the contacts that Thunberg had maintained between Uppsala and Edo. As Siebold sat in his study in the old monastery on the Rhine each morning, and later at Bonn, writing his memoirs of Japan, his thoughts constantly strayed to Nagasaki and Edo. He was still in his heart the great *sensei* of Japan, dedicated above all to the opening of the empire under circumstances which would not destroy the country and the culture that he loved so dearly.

Beyond his deep emotional bonds with Japan, it seems clear that Siebold understood the economic and cultural potential of the empire as a member of the world community. The enthusiasm with which his collections representing the arts, the horticulture, and the way of life of the Japanese had been received in Europe assured him of the important contributions that lay in those fields. The reliability, the capacity for hard work, and the skill of the Japanese indicated that Japan could as well become an important economic power.

五

V

The Continuing Rise of Western Medicine:
The Return of Siebold

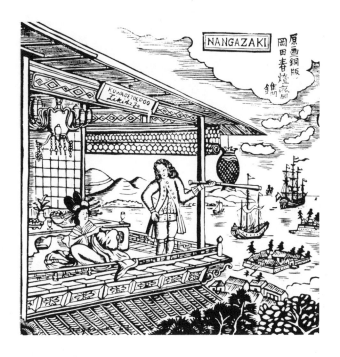

WESTERN MEDICINE CONTINUED to hold the center of the stage after Siebold's departure from Japan. Its unique role has been emphasized by Sir George Sansom:

> One of the remarkable features of Western studies in the pre-Restoration period was the great attention paid to surgery and medicine. A scholar named Ogata Kōan is said to have taught more than three thousand students in his school . . . in the twenty years before 1862, and there were many other private schools, all teaching Western medical and surgical methods and related subjects. From medical science it was only a short step to pharmacology, chemistry, and related subjects. Thus it will be seen that by 1868 the country was by no means unprepared for a further development of education on Western lines [1962, p. 451].

The translation of Western texts in astronomy, chemistry, physics, metallurgy, mathematics, navigation, and geography, as well as in medicine, continued to be a major activity of the *Rangakusha*.

The increasing importance of *Rangaku* led to mounting opposition by the Neo-Confucianists and the *bakufu*. Their anxieties were heightened by the rapidly crumbling social and economic structure of the feudal society as well as by the intrusions of foreign flags seeking diplomatic relations.

In response to the reactionary opposition, schools of Western medicine posted strict rules of conduct to protect their students. Representative of these are the regulations that were posted at Kyūrido in Kyoto by Koishi Genzui:

1. As for Dutch books, do not read any other books than medical books.

2. Do not slander people without giving any clear reason.

3. When there is no other appropriate translation available, it will be all right to use Dutch words (such as names of drugs, medical and surgical tools, and scientific signs and measurements), but otherwise do not write Dutch words, but use Japanese words.

4. Do not discuss subjects other than medicine when talking about foreign countries.

5. Also do not express foreign opinions, or carry or possess unusual tools [translated from Sekiuma, pp. 172–73].

The number of students entering the schools of Western medicine now far exceeded the limit that could be handled effectively by the teachers. The problem was compounded by the fact that the teachers were busy practitioners and relied in part on their earnings in practice to maintain the schools. One of the first to face this problem was Itō Genboku, who founded Shōsendō in Edo in 1834. After Shōsendō had been in operation for a few months, Ito concentrated his instruction on the first students to enroll. In turn he assigned the education of the stream of students who continued to enter the school to the older students. This resulted in a rather complicated arrangement for paying tuition fees to Itō in the traditional manner—in a sealed envelope accompanied by a fan in a highly polished lacquer box as a sign of respect. Upon entry every new student was also required to present minor fees to each of the older students who would serve as his teachers. An additional source of revenue for Itō came through the rule that the students must purchase all of their school supplies from him, and rice-paper handkerchiefs, always an essential part of their attire, from his wife.

Itō Genboku, a man of vision, was one of the first voices to speak out in criticism of the rigid hereditary pattern of entry into the medical profession. From his youth, the oldest son of a Japanese physician knew by unspoken tradition that he would not only serve as his father's apprentice but in due course succeed his father when he retired. Because a son was required to follow his father's dictates on all matters, this meant to Itō that Japanese medicine would continue rigid and unchanging for future generations. A son could not question or interpret the dogma that had been expounded by his father. Unfortunately, Itō's voice was not heeded, and, although the apprentice system disappeared, the strong tradition of the oldest son studying medicine and subsequently assuming his father's practice continues unchanged today.

The years with Siebold brought home to Itō Genboku the importance of practical clinical training in medicine; the skills of Western medicine could not be acquired by simply poring over Dutch texts. He realized that study under European physicians was essential but would be adopted only through public endorsement by the *bakufu*.

Itō's repeated requests for such endorsement were finally heeded in 1861 when the *bakufu* sent two of his students, Itō Gempaku and Hayashi Kenkai to Nagasaki. They enrolled in a medical school that had been established two years earlier by a young Hollander, Pompe van Meerdervoort (see Chapter VI). The following June the *bakufu* awarded scholarships to Itō and Hayashi to continue the study of medicine at The Hague. They were among the first Japanese students to receive governmental subsidy for further studies in Europe.

Another school for Western medicine, Wada Juku, was opened at Yagenbori in Edo in 1838 by Satō Taizen. He had considered studying medicine with Takano Chōei, but Takano was much too busy arguing national affairs and drinking sake to concern himself with teaching medicine. Satō Taizen studied at Nagasaki and Deshima with Narabayashi Eiken and J. F. Niemann for three years, 1835–38. On his return to Edo he opened Wada Juku. In 1843 the school moved from Edo to Sakura, in part as a precautionary measure because of Satō's relationship with the fugitive Takano Chōei. At Sakura, in the same year, he built a hospital which he named Juntendō, meaning "obey the way of heaven." The hospital gained fame through its pioneering efforts in the introduction of Western surgical techniques, especially in urological surgery.

Satō Taizen was one of the first Japanese physicians to use vaccination against smallpox and in this he antedated the introduction of lymph through Deshima.

Of the hospitals established to teach Western medicine during *Rangaku*, Juntendō is the only one which exists today under the same name. The Juntendō Medical School and Hospital stand today near O-cha-no-mizu ("tea water station") in Tokyo.

The leading role of Western medicine was enhanced in 1840 when the *bakufu* outlawed all Western studies except medicine.

As a result, the expanding body of students dedicated to all fields of Western learning turned to the schools of the teachers of medicine and surgery. The intensity of the official hostility against all Western studies except medicine has been commented on by Sansom: "It was dangerous for those who resided in Bakufu domains to display an interest in other branches of Western science" (1962, p. 257).

The opposition of the Neo-Confucianist doctors reached such heights that in 1849 the *bakufu* issued a special order forbidding the practice of Dutch medicine. However, in an interesting qualification, surgery and ophthalmology were not barred, because these fields were so popular and because the results of treatment were so readily observable that there could be no hidden adverse effects. The order was never strictly enforced; there were influential persons in the *bakufu* who were well aware of the value of Dutch medicine.

After 1840, as the medical schools enrolled students who sought instruction in physics, chemistry, and mathematics as well as in medicine and Dutch, the schools became institutes of science and technology, as well as of medicine. At this juncture such an institution in Osaka emerged to enduring national fame. Its master was the greatest teacher of the *Rangakusha*, Ogata Kōan.

Ogata Kōan was a singular inspiration to his students and is widely revered in Japan today as the perfect exemplar of scholarship, dedication, and rectitude, those attributes which the Japanese have through the centuries considered essential to the true teacher. He began the study of medicine at the age of fifteen in Osaka and after four years went to Nagasaki and then to Edo where he studied with Itō Genboku. After thirteen years as a student, Ogata Kōan returned to Osaka where in 1838 he entered the practice of medicine and established a small school. It was named Tekiteki-sai Juku; Teki was one of Ogata's pseudonyms. The school was destined to gain enduring fame, not only for the peerless qualities of its founder, but as well for the outstanding students who enrolled from across Japan. One of them, Fukuzawa Yukichi, was a leader in steering Japan to the road of intensive westernization. Another, Nagayo Sensai, was the first director of the Imperial Sanitary Bureau.

When Ogata Kōan opened Teki-juku he was young, he was poor, and he suffered from constant ill health due to a tuberculous lesion which was ultimately fatal. Despite his precarious health, Ogata set a grueling daily schedule. After many hours in the practice of medicine he would return to Teki-juku to present lectures to his students, to answer their questions, to befriend them, and to inspire them to a matchless zeal in their studies.

The zeal of Ogata Kōan's students was unmatched; at times they would study around the clock to master Dutch, Western medicine, and the rudiments of physics, chemistry, and biology. Since only a handful of texts were available, they were in constant use, and the students seized every opportunity to read and copy other books on Western science and technology. On one occasion, Ogata Kōan showed a group of students a Dutch text on electricity which he had borrowed, and their entreaties were so moving that he permitted them to keep the book for three days. They stayed at their desks without sleep and with just a snatch of food for two days and nights to copy the most important chapter. The only space that a student could call his own was the single *tatami* mat that served as his study hall, his recreation room, and his bedchamber.

Fortunately, both Fukuzawa Yukichi and Nagayo Sensai have left detailed descriptions of life at Teki-juku. Fukuzawa's autobiography is the standard reference to Teki-juku; it has been translated into English and widely quoted. Nagayo Sensai paints an equally vivid picture of life at the school:

I, Nagayo Sensai . . . entered under Ogata Kōan *sensei*, in June, 1854, and after the entrance ceremonies, lived in the *juku* in Kitahama. This *juku* was called Teki-juku and there were constantly more than 100 students from all over Japan. Its *rinkō* ("reading and explaining class") was in almost constant session and Teki-juku was considered the leading *juku* for Dutch studies in those days in the entire country. For *rinkō* students were divided into eight classes and each class had its examinations six times a month. The order of seats for those sessions was decided by drawing lots; the first student read and explained the first few lines of a Dutch book and the next student asked questions, and thus we took turns until the last student. For each question, Kaitō decided the winner and the loser, and gave a white mark to the winner and a black mark to the loser. "Kaitō" was shared among *juku* head, *juku* superviser, and

Ik'kyūsei ("advanced") students, depending on the advancement of the particular class.

When the first student finished his *rinkō* assignments, the class was dismissed. The marks accumulated during one month were checked and those who had the highest marks became the top students of the class, and the order of seats was changed accordingly every month.

The student who occupied the top seat consecutively advanced to the upper class. In the *juku*, each student was given one *tatami*-mat space for his own use, and as he had to put his desk, bedding, and other personal belongings in this space, and sleep and study there, it was extremely crowded. Especially those who had mats close to the entrance or facing the wall had to suffer, as they were stepped on during the night while they were sleeping or had to read by candlelight even during the day. And every month these spaces were changed according to the order of seats in the *rinkō*, and as those in the upper seats in the class could choose first the space they wanted, anyone who won even one point got the better living space from the next in line. Therefore, to win or to lose in the *rinkō* was extremely important for each student, but there were no sneaky students who would secretly ask help from others even for one word or one phrase, and thus each student using a dictionary translated on his own, and tested his ability with his own ingenuity. Students in the beginners' class were allowed to attend others' lectures and do *rinkō* freely, but most of the time students in the same class assembled and listened to lectures given by the advanced students.

The books used for *rinkō* were in the possession of the head of the *juku* and they were the only available copies. First, students in the same class copied them in turn and then started their preparatory readings.

In the beginning you did not know any words except articles and prepositions, and therefore it was necessary to use a dictionary for almost every word, but there was only one copy of a dictionary called "Zufu"— a Dutch-Japanese dictionary (a person by the name of "Zufu" came to Nagasaki and added Japanese meanings to a Dutch dictionary by François Halma)—in the entire *juku*. The room, the size of three *jō* ("mats") was called "Zufu" room and the dictionary was kept in the room and we were never allowed to take it out of the room.

As the more than one hundred students in the entire *juku* had to rely on this single copy of the dictionary, the room was constantly occupied by these students, who came in and out in turn and used the dictionary, pulling it to left and right, to front and back, and it was almost impossible to even touch it. As it was so hard to use the dictionary and find out the meaning of a word during the daytime, there were many who went to use it in the middle of the night when there were not many students in the room. Thus the light in the "Zufu" room was on throughout the night all year around. In those days, students used to say that if they could read Dutch books with a dictionary on their right hand, it would be the most pleasant thing in the whole world . . . [translated from Nagayo, pp. 3–5].

A second resource for the students in their study of Dutch was the *Nederduitsch Taalkundug Woordenboek* of P. Weiland. Since it was entirely in Dutch, it was of value only to the advanced students; for all others Doeff-Halma was the sole resource.

A knowledge of Dutch had now reached such importance that the feudal lords sought copies of Doeff's dictionary. They asked the advanced students at Teki-juku to edit parts of the dictionary for them and these opportunities afforded a tidy extra income for the students. The fee for writing a page of Dutch letters was twice the fee for writing a page of Japanese characters. When the lords spent the required months in residence at their palaces in Edo, they obtained copies of Doeff from students of *Rangaku* in the capital city. Fukuzawa tells of a student who made sufficient funds from this work to finance his education in Teki-juku. He expressed pointedly the attitude of students in Edo toward the importance of being able to study with Ogata Kōan: "Edo was a good place to make a living, but as for real study, it could not be done except in Osaka" (1960, p. 84).

A towering inspiration to his students, an imaginative teacher, and a gifted physician, Ogata Kōan had a singular affection for his students. When Fukuzawa Yukichi fell ill with typhoid fever, Ogata's personal distress was so deep that he declined to accept the full responsibility as "the chief" physician. He told Fukuzawa: "I will come every day to see you and give you as much advice as possible. But I am going to ask some other doctor to direct the use of medicine, because when a doctor knows his patients too well, he is apt to be anxious and do too many things, trying one medicine after another, and then suddenly remembering some other medicine, giving that too; and in that way he may miss what should be the proper treatment" (*ibid.*, p. 39). It is easy to understand why Fukuzawa could write in his diary: "the relation between teacher and student . . . was of the intimate, father-and-son kind. . . . when I was in Ogata's school, I could not but feel that I was a member of his family" (*ibid.*, pp. 40–41).

In addition to his contributions as a teacher and a physician, Ogata was the author of several important medical texts. He wrote the first Japanese text on general pathology and internal medicine, *Byōgaku Tsūron*, published in 1847–49 in twelve volumes. It consisted primarily of abstracts that had been translated from the writings of European physicians led by Christian Wilhelm Hufeland. Another important publication by Ogata Kōan was *Fushi keikun ikun*, a translation of part of Hufeland's *Enchiridion medicum* (Berlin, 1833), from the Dutch edition by Hageman (Amsterdam, 1838). Ogata translated the section entitled "Praxis." It was the first book published in Japanese describing in detail the physical examination of the chest and therefore was of distinct value because of the high incidence of pulmonary tuberculosis.

Ogata was called to Edo in 1862 to take the post of director of the Institute for Western Medicine. Just one year later, Fukuzawa, upon his return to Edo, received the sad news that his beloved teacher, physician, and spiritual father was coughing blood; he ran to Ogata's home only to find him dead. A final testament to the stature of this great teacher came at the time of his death through the continuing affection and loyalty of his students at his wake: "Some of his pupils who lived nearby were already there; others kept coming in. The small house was soon filled with forty or fifty men who overflowed from the parlor into the entrance hall. That night we were to sit up for the last watch over our old master" (*ibid.*, p. 158).

The frame building of Tekiteki-sai Juku has been restored in Osaka today. After crossing the *genkan*, the visitor sees on the other side of a small enclosed garden a bust of Ogata; the gentle, thoughtful countenance is the embodiment of the reverence felt by his pupils. He seems to greet the visitor as one of his pupils. On the second floor is the map room where the students fought for the Dutch-Japanese dictionary, and nearby the dormitory room where they huddled on their *tatami* mats by candlelight to work through the night writing Dutch or studying medicine, chemistry, or physics.

Fukuzawa Yukichi was a member of the first mission from Japan to the West. The progressive attitudes that were nurtured by his relationship with Ogata Kōan were influential in his decision to establish a school, Keio-gijuku, in Edo. From this developed Keio University; when classes opened in 1890, the first professors were three American scholars in law, literature, and economics who had been made available through the interest of President Charles W. Eliot of Harvard.

Ogata Kōan, if alive today, would take special pleasure in the splendid medical school that has developed at the university founded by Fukuzawa. The first dean was Kitasato Shibasaburō, one of the world's most distinguished bacteriologists, the first scientist to identify the plague bacillus, and as well a pioneer in elucidating the immune mechanism through his studies on tetanus. Keio was the first Japanese medical school to have visiting professors in residence from the United States and is today considered by many to be the leading medical school in Japan and the one with the strongest American orientation.

Today the simple frame building of Teki-juku in Osaka stands in sharp contrast to the splendid new Keio University Medical Center in Tokyo, one of Asia's leading teaching hospitals—the one the home of the teacher, the other the vision of his most renowned student. They symbolize the striking changes that have occurred in medicine in Japan in one century because of the influence and vision of a few great *Rangakusha*, of whom Ogata Kōan was one of the true leaders.

One year after the opening of Teki-juku another school of Western medicine was established in a picturesque setting in nearby Kyoto. It was located in a lovely garden by the massive gate of Nanzenji Temple at the foot of the verdant Higashiyama ("eastern mountains"). The founder, Shingū Ryōtei (1787–1854), from the fishing village Maizuru on the Japan Sea, studied in Nagasaki from October, 1813, until the spring of 1818. At the age of thirty-two, stimulated by the writings of Udagawa Genzui, he returned to Kyoto penniless but determined to open a medical school. He quickly established an excellent reputation as a practitioner of Western medicine to a degree that he was invited by several *daimyō* in the region to move to their courts as official

148

physician. But his determination to teach Western medicine prevailed. After twenty years in the practice of medicine, in 1839 Shingū accumulated sufficient funds to build Junsei-shoin, which in due course included a classroom, a library, and a dormitory reserved for the use of students in financial need. At the rear of the buildings he established a garden for the cultivation of medicinal plants. The curriculum, representative of that period, included lectures and demonstrations on anatomy, physiology, pathophysiology, natural history, materia medica, pathology, internal medicine, and surgery. As had Ōtsuki Gentaku, Shingū Ryōtei endeavored to advance the prestige of Western medicine but without discarding Japanese traditions. Shingū lectured on Chinese medicine, and a Confucian scholar lectured on Chinese classics and Chinese history three times a month.

Eighty years after the founding of Junsei-shoin, Sekiba Fujihiko visited the buildings of the school and left an interesting historical note:

On April 6, 1919, I (i.e., Sekiba) had occasion to visit my friend Dr. Watsuji Shunji at this Junsei-shoin in Kyoto. The part of the main building facing the fence of the Nanzenji Temple was the auditorium and in this there was a *tokonoma* ("alcove") of nine *shaku* ("Japanese foot") with a slightly raised seat in front of this *tokonoma*. The lecturer who taught Confucian classics sat on this seat and gave lectures.

In the days when Ryōtei was still living, it is said that a scroll of Confucius' teachings was hung in the *tokonoma*, and in another room there was hung a scroll of Shen Nung (Chinese medicine god). The frame hung on the wall had four characters written by Mabe Shodo, the governor in those days.

It was said that there were a fairly large number of Chinese and Dutch medical books, and Chinese classics and history books in the library, but now it is said that some of them were kept at the house of the Shingū family, and some were scattered after the Meiji Restoration.

The dormitory was used mainly to provide housing as assistance to the students who were financially poor. The rules of the dormitory were very liberal as the chief objective of this *juku* was a complete medical education, not merely translating Dutch books [translated from Sekiuma, 2: 189–90].

Four remarkable Japanese physicians and scholars—Sugita Gempaku, Maeno Ryōtaku, Ōtsuki Gentaku, and Ogata Kōan—were the leaders of *Rangaku*. They shared common characteristics: passion for scholarship, vision, and intellectual patriotism. They were determined that the geographical isolation of their country should not result in intellectual isolation.

Sugita Gempaku and Maeno Ryōtaku may be considered as the founders of *Rangaku*. The translation of the *Kaitai Shinsho* was a symbol to their followers. It was not the book itself that was significant; it was the two men who stood behind it. *Kaitai Shinsho* had a limited circulation, there were many errors, and the wood-block prints did not afford the clarity of detail desirable for an anatomical text. But the publication of the book in 1774 was the culmination of three years of intensive work by respected scholars. Their efforts were followed closely by students in Edo and Nagasaki who were watching to see if the "impossible" could be accomplished. It was not unlike an effort to scale Mount Everest in which each day's progress is followed by national news media; when the successful expedition has shown that it can be done, other expeditions follow, confident of success. So the publication of *Kaitai Shinsho* proved that it could be done, and soon other students turned to the study of Western medicine.

Fortunately, Sugita and Maeno did not close their books and turn back to the practice of medicine after the publication of *Kaitai Shinsho*. Instead, they became teachers of Dutch, Western medicine, and natural history; they took it to be their responsibility to do so. As teachers, as students, and as individuals, Sugita and Maeno were an ideal pair. They shared high intelligence and dedication to scholarship. Sugita was by nature a leader; Maeno was retiring and introspective. Sugita was ambitious; Maeno was self-effacing. Sugita was a generalist; Maeno concentrated on the study of the Dutch language. Ōtsuki Gentaku, attracted to Edo by their reputations as teachers, first studied with Sugita, who then sent him to Maeno because of the latter's greater knowledge of Dutch and Dutch science.

When Ōtsuki Gentaku came to Edo to study with Maeno and Sugita he assured the fulfillment of *Rangaku*. He took it as one of his major responsibilities to establish *Rangaku* as the most important field for Japanese students; through his remarkable flow of manuscripts, his teachings, and even his "Dutch New Year" he was successful. Ōtsuki fixed the eyes of Japanese students and scholars on Holland and Europe instead of China.

While Ōtsuki Gentaku was the leader of *Rangaku* in the Kantō area, Ogata Kōan was its leader in the Kansai area.

Ogata Kōan was the greatest teacher of the *Rangakusha* and gave new and vital impetus to *Rangaku* when he opened Teki-juku, eleven years after the death of Ōtsuki. Because of the repressive measures of the *bakufu*, he attracted students of wide interests and abilities who were leaders in the final and official adoption of Western influences.

Siebold's Return to Japan

Philipp Franz von Siebold's long cherished dream to return to Japan became a reality when he arrived at Nagasaki on August 14, 1859. He was destined for a second cycle of deep satisfaction culminating in disappointment, bitterness, and another forced departure from the land that he loved. And for a second time his problems were due in large part to his driving ambition. On his first visit he had been determined to be a scientific conqueror; on his second visit he was determined to be a diplomatic conqueror. There was hardly a role less suited for Siebold than that of a diplomat, and the circumstances could hardly have been less favorable. With complete confidence he assumed a responsibility which a King Solomon or a Prince Metternich would have found impossible.

For two decades Siebold waged an intensive campaign to find a country that would open the empire and send him back to Japan. His first approach was to The Netherlands, and in his role as adviser to The Hague he repeatedly urged William II to make a direct appeal to the shogun. On February 15, 1844, the king affixed his signature and the royal seal to a letter drafted in part by Siebold and addressed to the shogun, Tokugawa Ieyoshi. The king advised the shogun of the rapidly changing relationships between the Orient and the West.* William II stated that China had been forced to open five ports to European nations

* See Appendix I of this volume for the letter and the shogun's reply.

and that in the attendant conflict thousands of Chinese had been killed, cities devastated, and millions in treasure seized by the conquerors. The king foresaw similar problems for Japan and quoted a Chinese philosopher, Lao-tzu: "When wisdom is seated on the throne, she will excel in maintaining peace." William II concluded with a recommendation:

> This, Allpowerful Emperor, is our friendly advice, ameliorate the laws against the foreigners, lest happy Japan be destroyed by war. We give Your Majesty this advice with honest intentions, free from political self-interest.
>
> We hope that wisdom will make the Japanese government realise that peace can only be maintained through friendly relations, and that these are only created by commercial relations.

In his reply the shogun acknowledged the gifts that the king had forwarded with his letter but stated that any amelioration of the laws against the foreigners "cannot be, as of now, through the inconvenience of the country." At the same time he assured William II that Dutch subjects would continue to be welcome to trade in Japan in the future and that the shogun would protect them in the same manner as his own subjects.

Four years later, in 1848, Siebold turned to Germany in his efforts to find a country that would launch an expedition to open Japan. He approached Archduke Johannes, a Hapsburg, who had been elected imperial vicar of the newly organized Frankfurt Assembly. But the fall of the assembly the following year as part of the power struggle that was sweeping Germany dashed Siebold's hopes that representatives of his fatherland would sail to the Orient.

In 1852 Siebold renewed his campaign to bring The Netherlands into the role of leadership in the opening of Japan. But William II had died in 1849 and his successor, William III, concentrated on commercial and other internal developments; he was not interested in expanding a colonial empire.

Stalled at The Hague, Siebold turned eastward to Russia as the country that should open Japan. His visit to St. Petersburg and Moscow in 1834 had made an indelible impression on Siebold; he held a lifelong respect for Russia. His approach to

St. Petersburg came at a time when Russia had become deeply interested in Japan, in part because of Japan's geographical proximity to Russia's Asian provinces. As early as 1739, and again in 1742, a Russian expedition had visited the coasts of Japan but had been turned away. In 1804 a Russian delegation had been rebuffed at Nagasaki.

In 1849 Count K. V. Nesselrode, the Russian foreign minister, determined that in order to thwart American and British interests in the Far East, Russia must be the first country to open Japan. Siebold learned of the Russian interest in Japan and sent an unsolicited communication to St. Petersburg in which he emphasized the importance of the proposed undertaking and advised on how it might be successful.

As Siebold turned his interests in the opening of Japan toward the East, more important developments were taking place in the West. They brought Siebold into an interesting but little-known relationship with the Perry expedition to open Japan. Siebold met his match in Commodore Perry, whose aggressiveness, self-assurance, and imperiousness were at least equal to those qualities in Siebold. The Commodore used Siebold's references and maps but absolutely refused to accept his offer to join the expedition.

In 1852 the Department of State and the Department of the Navy in Washington jointly decided to implement a resolution of 1846 and organize an expedition to Japan. On January 27, 1852, Secretary of State Daniel Webster sent a dispatch to the U.S. chargé d'affaires at The Hague, George Folsom, directing him to obtain from the Dutch any maps, charts, or other information on Japan which would be useful for the expedition. In conformity with their historic agreement with the Japanese, the Hollanders sent a special report to Edo advising the *bakufu* of this development.

The first collection of material from the Dutch which Folsom forwarded to Secretary Webster included "copies of the maps attached to the latest great work upon Japan, that of Siebold, who went out in 1823 as physician to the Dutch Factory and remained there several years in that capacity" (Record Group 59, National Archives). The alarm raised in Edo by the proposed expedition was evident in the same note: "According to advices from the Indies which, however, need confirmation, the Court of Jedo, relying upon ancient treaties, has invited the aid of The Netherlands in case of an invasion from the United States."

The requests from Washington for information on Japan placed the Hollanders in an awkward position. They were naturally disturbed at the thought of another and more powerful nation moving toward the key role in opening Japan to the world after they had endured the humiliations at Deshima and Edo for more than two centuries. The Americans continued to seek Dutch support and went as far as to request The Hague to order the *opperhoofd* at Deshima to lend all possible assistance to the expedition in the hope that this would assure that there would be no military action. But the Dutch had determined that they would do nothing significant to assist the United States. They refused to take any steps that might compromise their relations with the court at Edo since they anticipated that the nation which endeavored to open the country would be drawn into armed combat with the Japanese. In the event of such a development the Hollanders believed that their status would be materially enhanced if they were on the side of the shogun rather than that of the invaders. They were willing to pass along to America manuscripts, maps, and charts which already were public property, but they would not consider any other support for the expedition.

Siebold learned of the impending expedition and the American requests for intelligence on Japan. Isolated in the old abbey at Boppard on the Rhine, he wanted desperately to know more about the expedition, to give advice, but above all to become a member of the group that would open Japan. He insisted on firsthand information and to obtain it took the most direct route—he invited George Folsom to visit him at Boppard.

The report by the American chargé d'affaires to Secretary Webster gives an interesting picture of Siebold living in another unique environment after his Japanese surroundings in Holland. Folsom found Siebold residing in an old nunnery:

Having received a pressing invitation from Col. Siebold to make him a visit at his residence on the Rhine, and wishing to place two of my children at school in Germany, I took passage from Rotterdam up the river immediately after sending off my despatch of the 20th ultimo. We proceeded as far as Neumied, a few miles below Coblentz, where having made arrangements for the school and leaving my family, I went up to Boppard and had the good fortune to find Siebold at home. He resides in a noble chateau, formerly the Abbey of St. Martin, situated a little above the town, within a stone's throw of the Rhine, and in the midst of some of the finest scenery on the river. The premises are quite interesting to one not familiar with the religious houses of the olden time, having undergone but slight changes in being adapted to the purposes of a family residence; the long corridors with numerous apartments opening upon them, cloistered vaults and passages below, the chapel and its slender turret, all bespeak the pious uses to which the building was originally consecrated. It was long the abode of religious women, but the French Revolution put an end to this as well as all other monastic institutions on the Rhine, and turned adrift the unfortunate inmates, who were treated in the most shocking manner by the sacrilegious Gauls. Not a few of them are said to have had the cares of maternity cast on their future lot, which is not difficult to believe when the character of French warfare is considered.

Since that period St. Martin has passed into private hands and was purchased a few years ago by Col. Siebold for the residence of his family. I found him busily engaged with the last sheets of his great work, and received a hearty welcome at his hands. This was the more kind of him, considering the humble character of his guest, as he had entertained a few weeks before no less a personage than the King of Prussia, who made him a visit during his sojourn at the Castle of Stalyenfels in the immediate neighborhood of Coblentz. Of course Siebold was indebted for this notice from royalty to his reputation as a savant, and the fame of his residence in Japan. Although a native of Prussia, he had early entered the science of Holland, from whose government he now enjoys a retiring pension with the rank of Colonel, to which he is entitled from his former position as a chief of the medical staff of the army; but his residence is within the jurisdiction of Prussia.

I was glad to find that Siebold with his superior knowledge of Japan had great confidence in the success of Commodore Perry's proposed visit to that Empire. Everything depends, however, he thinks, on the political skill employed in the negotiation with the Japanese government, the use of mere force not being likely to produce the desired result. But the Japanese are so peculiar in their ideas, that there will be great difficulty in coming to an understanding with them without more than ordinary tact, which those who have been conversant with their habits and character are of course the most competent to bring into play. I have no doubt that Siebold himself would be of great service to the expedition, were he to accompany Commodore Perry, and should you desire to avail of his intimate knowledge of the country, of the government and of the character of the people, I am authorized to make a tender of his services to you. He consents to this with the hope that, if his offer should be accepted, he may be able to contribute to the success of an enterprise which he regards as one of the most important that can employ the energy of a great nation. I therefore submit to your consideration his proposal to accompany the expedition in which capacity as you may think proper.

Siebold's book is now quite completed and he intends to ask our government to request a copy, which he will forward to Washington as soon as possible. The price and worth is necessarily so high as to deter individuals of moderate means from pursuing it; but Holland as well as other European governments have encouraged the publication by subscribing for a number of copies. The King of Prussia has taken ten copies, Russia I believe the same number [Folsom to Webster, 6 August 1852, Record Group 59, National Archives].

Neither Siebold's offer of his services to Folsom nor a subsequent offer directly to Perry was ever acknowledged.

Five months after his conference with Folsom and still hopeful that he would be invited to join the Perry expedition, Siebold on January 9, 1853, received an invitation from Czar Nicholas I to visit St. Petersburg. Siebold felt no hesitation in recording in his diary that the Russian court sought "To get information from me personally on a certain matter, which no other European would have been able to give them" (1854, p. 5).

A few months earlier the czar had ordered that preparations be made for an expedition to Japan under Admiral E. V. Putyatin. Siebold's advice was sought on the expedition, on territories in the Kurile Islands, and on the Amur River boundaries which had been disputed with China since 1689. At Siebold's suggestion the czar sent a letter to the shogun urging the settlement of any boundary questions in the northern islands and the opening of ports to Russian trade. In recognition of his services the czar conferred the rank of Commander des Vlad mir-ordens on Siebold.

The trip to Russia was the last nail in the coffin that bore Siebold's dreams of becoming a member of the Perry expedition. On March 8, 1853, George Folsom informed Edward Everett, who had succeeded Webster as secretary of state, that Siebold had gone to St. Petersburg at the invitation of the czar, who wished to consult him about a proposed Russian expedition to Japan. American Russophobia was decisive, and the official narrative of the expedition states the basis for Perry's rejection of Siebold's services: "on personal grounds since from information received from abroad he suspected von Siebold of being a Russian spy and he knew that he had been banished" (Hawks, p. 79).

Siebold was embittered and only added fuel to the fire when he ascribed the opening of Japan to the Russians, not to the Americans, in a pamphlet that he published at Bonn in 1854. This drew a sharp rebuttal from the expedition, and Siebold was described as "the self-constituted court chamberlain of Japan" (*ibid.*).

Perry used Siebold's charts in navigating Japanese waters and his books for vital information on Japan. There are several references to Siebold's reports in the official narrative of the expedition. The legend of the major map of Japan in this document reads: "Map of the Japan Islands copied from Von Siebold's with slight additions and corrections, by the U.S. Japan Expedition and other authorities. Compiled by order of Commodore M. C. Perry, U.S.N., by Lieuts, W. L. Maury and Silas Bent, 1855" (*ibid.*, pp. 126–27).

Perry was quite willing to blame Siebold when one of the expedition's ships, the U.S.S. *Macedonian*, ran aground in Japanese waters. The inaccurate chart was described as "nothing more than a copy of one of von Siebold's maps" (*ibid.*, p. 326).

Siebold was decidedly better off nursing his grudges at Bonn than he would have been as a member of the Perry expedition. The Commodore and Siebold simply could not have tolerated each other; the domineering attitude that they shared would have brought them into direct conflict in short order. One would have fallen—and since Siebold could not topple a Commodore, he would have been the casualty.

To facilitate his communications with heads of state and to enjoy the intellectual life of a university town, Siebold moved to Bonn at the end of 1853. He joined a discussion group, and the chronicles of its meetings include descriptions of the conferences held at Siebold's residence. In the first discussion Siebold pointed out the passion of the Japanese for foreign knowledge; he also deliberately re-created the frigid temperatures of a Japanese home in the winter months:

No. 161—7 February 1857—*von Siebold*.
It was so cold in the room that one's fingers became stiff. Cigars were not passed around.
The lecture dealt with the literature and geographical knowledge of Japan. Many old and new works were exhibited. The Japanese thirst for knowledge is very large. In contrast to the Chinese, they have an interest in everything that is foreign, although they try to keep foreigners at a distance. The musical dramatic presentations in which the female roles are taken by the other sex are impressive. One went down stairs for food— into a somewhat warmer room in which one began to recover [translated from Naumann].

At another discussion Siebold displayed his wide range of knowledge on oriental subjects:

No. 169—4 April 1857—*von Siebold*.
At tea the same member talked to us again around his large mahogany table, which he held to be a unique work. Afterward he presented no formal lecture, but instead talked about the devastating effects of the typhoons, the well-known cyclonic hurricanes of the China Sea. Here he cited several examples of the calm outside the edge of the vortex. Then the same member touched on all sorts of unique aspects of Japanese mining and medicine. These comments were illustrated by means of pictures. The discussion about Japan was continued at the dining table [*ibid.*].

At the third meeting Siebold's desire to impress his colleagues seems to have carried him into historical fantasies:

No. 177—20 February 1858—*von Siebold*.
For the first time cigars were offered, which resulted in a certain satisfaction. The lecturer appeared, in my opinion, to

be trying to prove a historical impossibility in that he proposed to establish the famous Atilla of the Middle Ages and world conqueror, Genghis Khan, as Japanese; he was said to be none other than Josizma, the brother of Joritzma, the first shogun or tycoon; in order to escape the persecution of his brother, Josizma is supposed to have gone across the seas to the Mongol tribe of Taotse; here he soon came into esteem, honor, and finally power, whereupon he decided as the "*Oberkhan*" to conquer the world. At the table, members tried to prove to the speaker that he had become an ultra-Japanese [*ibid.*].

The bitterness engendered by Perry's rebuff and the success of the expedition intensified Siebold's determination to return to Japan. He turned again to The Hague and asked the Hollanders to send him to Nagasaki. On December 5, 1855, Mr. Donker Curtius, the Dutch consul and *opperhoofd* at Nagasaki, officially requested the Nagasaki *bugyō* to have the sentence of lifelong banishment revoked. The *bakufu*, now deeply involved with the West and eager to hold the support of the Dutch, lifted the ban. More than three years were to elapse before Siebold once again sailed into Nagasaki Bay. A treaty establishing full diplomatic relations between the Dutch and the Japanese was not ratified until August 18, 1858. Another factor in the delay was the reluctance of the Dutch to allow a former exile to return to Japan under their auspices.

Undaunted, Siebold decided to use personal funds for the trip. However, the Nederlandsche Handels-Maatschapij, successor to the Dutch East India Company, appointed him adviser to their agency in Nagasaki and supported his passage to Japan. In April, 1859, Siebold, accompanied by his thirteen-year-old son Alexander, left Bonn on the first leg of his long-awaited return trip to Japan.

On his departure Siebold received a heart-warming farewell message from Baron Alexander von Humboldt (translated from P. F. von Siebold, 1897, pp. 251–52):

It is for the older traveler to express publicly how much he admires my dear and illustrious confrere, a resolution nobly inspired by the same dedication for the sciences which was

159

carried forward for a half century by your rare activity and the variety of your knowledge which has born such eminent fruit.

There is no aspect of physical geography which has not profited from your immense works regarding the archipelago of Japan. Our botanical gardens are decorated with plants that you have introduced. You are going to the same places again to continue and perfect these magnificent works. May your health, which is so dear to all those who take an interest in the progress of physical sciences, hold up under this new undertaking so that you may fulfill the wishes of your old and affectionate friends and admirers.

Berlin, April 10, 1859   s/Alexander de Humboldt

After extensive discussions of the political and economic events in Japan with officials at Batavia, Siebold, with Alexander at his side, sailed into Nagasaki Bay on August 14, 1859, thirty years after his expulsion. His memories were bittersweet; he was eager to see his daughter Ine, to renew his studies, and hopefully to become embroiled in the tumultuous events in Edo. Typically his luggage included six hundred and seventy-eight books, principally on voyages of discovery and descriptions of oriental and African countries and the Americas.

The reunion with O-Taki-san was less than happy. The once beautiful geisha and devoted wife had married on two occasions and was hawking kerosene on the streets of Nagasaki. But the reunion with O-Ine was a delight. Now thirty-one years old, she had studied with several of Siebold's former students and, pursuing the historic Siebold interest in obstetrics, had established herself as a leading midwife in Nagasaki. She was married to Ishii Sōken, one of Siebold's former students.

Siebold immediately perceived the strong animosity between the Japanese and the foreigners in Nagasaki; he found the aggressive attitudes of the British and the Americans especially distressing. And he was saddened by what he considered to be the beginning of the disappearance of the Japanese customs and traditions that he loved.

He temporarily established his residence in an old Buddhist temple, Honrenji, at the foot of the hill where the Christian martyrs were crucified in the sixteenth century. Many residents of Nagasaki recognized and acclaimed the tall, bearded figure who had walked their streets thirty years earlier. At first Siebold was reluctant to accede to the requests that he resume his former role as teacher and physician; he had been away from medicine for many years. But soon he relented and taught and practiced medicine at Honrenji.

Yet Siebold's eyes were on Edo, which was now the center of the struggle between the reactionaries, who wished to cling to the closed country, and the progressive forces, who were determined to open Japan. The problems were compounded by the embassies of Western Europe aggressively seeking favorable treaties for trade. They drew the bitter antagonism of the reactionary forces. The shogunate was crumbling. The hostility toward foreigners was intense in Nagasaki, and when Siebold went out to attend his patients in the evening, a bodyguard of servants marched in front, at his side, and behind him, waving aloft large lanterns on which were printed the characters representing the name of the famous doctor.

In April, 1860, George Smith, D.D., the bishop of Victoria, British crown colony of Hong Kong, came to Nagasaki. He was aware of Siebold's reputation as an authority on Japan and visited him at Honrenji. He found Siebold's relations with the Japanese to be excellent: "Any prejudice excited against the colonel by portions of his former history appears to have passed away. . . . He and his son . . . were everywhere welcomed by the Japanese in the neighbouring temples, and appeared to be regarded as favourites and well-known friends" (Smith, pp. 209–10). And Siebold was an invaluable source of information for the bishop, who was impressed with his easy friendship with the Buddhist priests and his facility in Japanese.

It was soon after the visit of Bishop Smith that Siebold moved into his old home on the beautiful hillside at Narutaki. A Nagasaki student, Takahashi, described Siebold in a familiar setting:

At the beginning of the *Bun-kyū* era, 1861, when I lived in Nagasaki to study the Dutch language, von Siebold came to Japan for the second time and lived with his little son Alexander in the village of Narutaki-mura. One day I started out to visit him. His house was surrounded by a large garden in which there were planted thousands of pharmaceutical plants and a wide variety of flowers. It was at the same time a geological garden, in which specimens of metals, rocks, etc., from our country had been collected, a very complete collection where nothing was missing. I saw von Siebold. He wore a beautiful beard, white as snow. He was a tall and handsome man with a distinguished appearance [translated from Kleiweg de Zwaan, p. 514].

With no inkling of the troubles that lay ahead, Siebold told the Prussian ambassador, Count Eulenburg, who visited him at Narutaki, that "he would never return to Europe . . . [that he was] in love with Japan and the Japanese and [would] complete his studies in Japan" (translated from Körner, p. 32). His reunion with Japan seemed complete.

One year after his arrival at Nagasaki the *bakufu* began to discuss the possibility of bringing Siebold to Edo as an adviser on foreign relations. Siebold had drawn their attention through a typical unsolicited communication from him in which he advised the *bakufu* not to accede to a request from the British and the French for permission to establish a base on the Japanese island of Tsushima off the coast of China. He warned that they wished to use it as a watchtower looking at China. In the same communication Siebold told the *bakufu* that his contract with the Nederlandsche Handel-Maatschapij would expire in April, 1861, and that he would be available to serve the government in Edo after that date. He transmitted another unsolicited letter of advice through official channels to the Dutch government. In this communication, which won him no friends, he stated that the exchange rate of sen for guldens was unfair to the Japanese and insisted that prompt action be taken by the Dutch to correct this injustice.

Siebold's former students Itō Genboku, Totsuka Seikai, and Takeuchi Gendō, aware of his hunger for fame, used their influence as physicians to the shogunate to support an invitation to Siebold. They felt that by helping their former teacher achieve his goal, they would be repaying some of the debt that they would carry for a lifetime as his former students.

On December 24, 1860, the *bakufu* forwarded a letter to Siebold through the Nagasaki *bugyō* to learn if he would respond favorably to an invitation to come to Edo as an adviser. The letter pointed out that his advice was needed on foreign affairs and on scientific and technical achievements in the West. When a delighted Siebold responded in the affirmative, he received an invitation to come to Edo with the official designation as adviser on Western science and technology. Foreign relations was considered to be too sensitive an area for public acknowledgment. It was understood, however, that Siebold's primary activities would be as adviser to the *bakufu* on foreign relations and political problems.

There could hardly have been a less propitious time to take on the role of political and international adviser to the government in Edo. Treaties had been signed with Russia, Holland, and England; and in July, 1858, a commercial treaty was signed with the United States. (In February, 1858, the shogunate sent two Japanese physicians trained in Dutch medicine to care for Townsend Harris, the U.S. consul general; they were directed to effect a cure or their lives would be in peril.) The door to Japan was open, but there were many Japanese who wished to slam it shut. "The cry of 'expel the barbarians' grew in all quarters of the land" (Reischauer, 1952, p. 111). In such a setting Philipp Franz von Siebold went to Edo to undertake what he envisaged as a major diplomatic responsibility for an embattled government. His dream of the role of a King Solomon or Prince Metternich was realized.

Siebold arrived at Yokohama on April 19, 1861, and remained there for two months. Tensions in Edo were so high that it was not until one month later that Takeuchi Shimotsuke-no-kami Yasunori, the foreign officer, and an associate, Kuwaji Saemonojō, felt that it was safe to consult Siebold. They proposed that a Japanese delegation visit the leading European powers, especially Britain and France, in an effort to persuade them to support Japan in a more Fabian course in opening her ports to trade. Siebold believed that this was desirable but was unsuccessful in his efforts to persuade a foreign power to make a ship available for such a mission.

Takeuchi also asked Siebold to send him a letter setting forth his terms of employment, and a manuscript copy of this communication is in the Kure Collection at the library of Tokyo University:

At Yokohama, May 27, 1861.
Presented at the feet of Edo Gaikoku Bugyō stationed here in Yokohama. . . . I should like to advise Japanese Government on the following points.

1. To smooth the trade relations between Japan and other foreign countries.

2. Give information and advice on governments of European countries.

3. Advise on Japanese products (materia medica, etc.) which might be suitable for export.

4. Advise on studies, agricultural techniques, and technical tools, etc.

5. Establish a Navy and enlarge it, educate officers and sailors. *

At the end of the letter Siebold pointed out that he had resigned his position as adviser to the Dutch trading company and inquired about his terms of employment with the *bakufu*, including salary, housing, and duration of employment.

On June 17, 1861, Siebold moved to Akabane, an official residence in Edo with a staff that included a director, a translator, and a secretary. Military guards were posted at the entry. Ten days later he agreed to a request from the *bakufu* that he open classes on Western science and military programs. However, in his reply he stated that his paramount wish was to advise on political and trade relations with the foreign powers. He emphasized that he considered these to be the most important problems and that he was prepared to instruct the high officials of the *Gaikoku* ("Foreign Office") on foreign relations. Siebold was disappointed when the reply, signed by all ranking members

* Zoku-Tsūshin zenran, Ranjin Shīboruto chōko ikken [On the case of hiring a Dutch person, Siebold], 1:20–23.

of the Foreign Office, stated that the situation was too sensitive for him to establish such a program and that he should concentrate on teaching Western science.

However, Siebold took every opportunity to involve himself as an adviser on foreign problems. He flooded the Foreign Office with memoranda on the sensitive relationships with the foreign embassies. Within a month, officials from the Foreign Office were coming to Siebold's office at Akabane for advice, and he began to visit the Foreign Office to discuss problems.

On several occasions Siebold placed himself in the most unwise position of serving as the appeaser for the *bakufu* against the foreign ambassadors. In the summer of 1861 a band of *rōnin* set fire to the British legation, and Siebold rushed to the scene to placate the angry British ambassador, Sir Rutherford Alcock. Siebold drew further hostility when Townsend Harris, the American consul, decided to remain in Edo while the other diplomats withdrew to Yokohama because of their concern for their safety and the inability of the Japanese government to control her citizens. The diplomats who moved to Yokohama were disturbed at Harris' insistence on remaining in Edo, and Siebold unwisely inserted himself into this troubled picture again to attempt the role of the unsolicited peacemaker. This was especially abrasive to the Dutch consul general, de Witt, because Siebold did not hesitate to refer to his long association with the Dutch. De Witt's anger was fanned when he learned that Siebold was writing unsolicited memoranda to the officials at Batavia for transmittal to The Hague. He then decided that Siebold's role as adviser to the *bakufu* and his meddling in the affairs of the foreign delegations must be stopped. The only way to accomplish this was to get Siebold out of Japan. There was strong sentiment that Siebold was trying to wear two hats—as representative of the *bakufu* and as representative of the Western powers. This could not be tolerated, especially when negotiations were so sensitive.

The Dutch consul general's first move was to suggest that Siebold leave Edo on the grounds that the Dutch government could not be responsible for his personal safety. Siebold countered by pointing out that he had military guards supplied by the *bakufu.* De Witt continued his protests and the pressure on the harried shogunate to discharge Siebold grew steadily. On December 17, 1861, a representative of the *bakufu*, Andō Tajima-no-kami, advised de Witt that they were releasing Siebold from their employ on that very day and that de Witt could then decide on Siebold's future in Japan. There was no question about the decision; de Witt was determined to rid Japan of Siebold. As a ruse Siebold was informed by de Witt that he had been appointed adviser on Japan to the governor at Batavia and that at a later date, when feelings in Edo had cooled, he would return to Edo as a representative of the Dutch government. Confident of an early return, Siebold left Alexander with an Englishman, Edward Clark, who arranged an appointment for the youth, now fifteen years old, as a supernumerary interpreter at the British legation.

Siebold's second trip to Japan was of little significance in the rise of Western medicine. The months in Nagasaki were rewarding for the reunion with Ine and with his former students. But the center of attraction in Nagasaki was no longer Siebold. It was a brilliant young Hollander, Pompe van Meerdervoort, who had established a new medical school which attracted students from across Japan. Siebold had no role in the program of the school, although in his diary Pompe commented on his contributions to medicine and science in Japan.

The effort to serve as adviser to the Foreign Office in Edo was a personal disaster. It passed unnoticed in the numerous diaries of that period, including those of Alcock and Harris. Thus for a second time Siebold sailed away from Nagasaki, embittered yet still in love with Japan.

When Siebold reached Batavia he soon realized that the post as adviser was simply a ruse, but his appeals to return to Nagasaki were of no avail. On the long voyage to Europe he laid his plans for one final campaign to return to Japan. His first hope lay in The Hague, but William III continued to concentrate on internal affairs and refused to be concerned with a tempest-in-a-teapot in far-off Japan. Siebold then turned to St. Petersburg with the hope that he might be able once again to stir an interest in the Far

East. But Russia had signed advantageous treaties with Japan in 1855, 1857, and 1858 and had no wish to become embroiled in a dispute with the shogunate.

Now thoroughly disillusioned, Siebold returned to his wife and children in Bonn. A promotion to the rank of major general in The Netherlands East Indies Army only poured salt on old wounds. On October 7, 1863, his resignation from that army was accepted with glowing statements lauding his contributions to the rise of the Dutch in the Far East.

Despite his disappointments, Siebold continued to hope for a third visit to Japan. His spirits rose in the fall of 1865 when Napoleon III summoned him to Paris for advice on a plan to establish a variety of relationships between France and Japan. The emperor, who envisaged a world-wide economic role for France, was interested in establishing a Franco-Japanese trading company, as well as a vocational school for teaching manual arts and a *lycée*. In the *lycée* Japanese youth would study French and French culture to prepare for enrollment at the University of Paris. Siebold developed a prospectus for the undertaking, but the idea of a government-sponsored company was strongly opposed by French capitalists. The opening of hostilities between Austria and Prussia, which threatened to engulf Europe, put an end to Louis Napoleon's plans.

Fortunately, during his period in Paris, Siebold developed a friendship with the popular French novelist Alphonse Daudet. Daudet has written a charming vignette of his association with Siebold, and of the circumstances surrounding the death of the old explorer, under the title "L'Empereur Aveugle ou Le Voyage en Baviere a la Recherche d'une Tragedie Japonaise" in *Contes du Lundi*. He brings out the heart-warming side of Siebold's personality—his eccentricities—and his unswerving love for Japan.

In the spring of 1866, M. de Sieboldt, Bavarian colonel in the service of Holland, well known in scientific circles for his beautiful works on Japanese flora, came to Paris to submit to the emperor a vast project of international scope for the exploitation of this marvelous *Nipon-Jepen-Japon* ("Empire of the Rising Sun") where he had lived for more than thirty years. While waiting for an audience at the Tuileries, the illustrious

167

traveler—still very Bavarian in spite of his stay in Japan—spent his evenings in a *brasserie* in the Poissonniere district in the company of a young lady from Munich who traveled with him, and whom he introduced as his niece. That is where I met him. The physiognomy of this grand old man, firm and straight as a rod in spite of his seventy-two years, his long white beard, his interminable greatcoat, his enribboned lapel where all the academies of sciences had put their colors, this strange air, a combination of timidity and lack of constraint, always made heads turn when he entered. Gravely the colonel sat down and pulled from his pocket a fat black radish; then the little young lady, very German in her short skirt, her fringed shawl, her small traveling hat, cut the radish into thin slices as was customary in her country, covered it with salt, offering it to her "ouncle" as she said it in her small mousy voice, and both, facing each other, began nibbling away quietly and simply, without questioning for a second that there could be anything ridiculous in doing in Paris as one does in Munich. They were truly a likable and original couple, and we soon became great friends. He, seeing how much I liked hearing him speak about Japan, had asked me to prod his memory, and I did not hesitate in accepting, as much out of friendship for this old Sinbad as for the purpose of burying myself in the study of the beauty of this country, a love for which he had communicated to me. This reviewing process was not unpainful. All the memories were written in the bizarre French that M. de Sieboldt spoke: "If I were to have shareholders, . . . if I could reunite the funds, . . . " and the vagaries of pronunciation which regularly made him say: "*le grandes boites de l'Asie*" for "*le grands poetes de l'Asie*," and "*Chabon*" for "*Japon*." With this, sentences that went on for fifty lines without a period, without a comma, leaving no time to breathe, yet so well organized in the mind of the author that to remove one word seemed impossible to him, and if I removed a line at some point, he would insert it at a later point. It was all the same! this devil of a man was so interesting with his "*Chabon*" that I forgot the tedium of work; and when that letter announcing the audience arrived, his memory was just about completely renewed.

Poor old Sieboldt! I can still see him walking toward the Tuileries, all his decorations on his chest, in his beautiful red and gold colonel's uniform that he pulled out of his trunk only for the grandest occasions. Whatever he made of it— "brum! brum!" all the time while straightening his long figure, to the trembling of his arm on mine, above all to the unusual paleness of his nose, a nice fat *nez de savantasse* crimsoned by study and Munich beer—I felt how moved he was. That evening, when I saw him, he was triumphant: Napoleon III had received him between two doors, listened to him for five minutes, and ended the audience with his favorite phrase: "I shall see. . . . I will think about it." On the basis of that, the naïve Japanese was all ready to rent a floor in the Grand Hotel, to write to the newspapers, to launch programs. I had a great deal of difficulty in making him understand that His Majesty might be quite long in thinking, and that in the meanwhile he would do best to return to Munich, where the Chamber was in the process of voting funds for the purchase of his great collection. My observations finally convinced him, and he left promising to send me, for my troubles with the famous memoire, a sixteenth-century Japanese tragedy entitled "The Blind Emperor," a precious masterpiece totally unknown in Europe which he had translated expressly for his friend Meyerbeer, who, at the time of his death, was composing music for the chorus. As you see, this was a real gift the good gentleman wished to offer me.

Unfortunately, several days after his departure, war broke out in Germany, and I heard no more of my tragedy. The Prussians having invaded Würtemberg and Bavaria, it is quite natural that in his patriotic fervor and the general disarray caused by an invasion, the colonel forgot my "Blind Emperor." But I was thinking about it more than ever, and, my goodness, in part wanting my Japanese tragedy, in part curious to see what war and invasion were at first hand—Oh God, the entire horror of this memory is with me now—I decided one fine day to leave for Munich.

It was in one of these harmonic cafes that I found Colonel Sieboldt, sitting with his niece, in front of his eternal black radish.

At the neighboring table, the minister of foreign affairs was having a stein of beer in the company of the king's uncle. All around, the good bourgeois families, officers with monocles, students with small caps in red, blue, sea green, all sullen (and) silent, religiously listening to the orchestra of M. Gungel and looked at the smoke rising from their pipes, no more concerned with Prussia, as if she did not exist at all. On seeing me, the colonel seemed uneasy, and I thought being aware of the fact, he lowered his voice to speak to me in French. Around us we heard whispered "Frenchmen . . . Frenchmen. . . ." "Let us leave," M. de Sieboldt said to me, and once outside, I found his old smile back. The good gentleman had not forgotten his promise, but he was very absorbed by

169

putting in order his Japanese collection that he had just sold to the state. That is why he had not written me. As for my tragedy, it was at Würtzburg in the hands of Madame de Sieboldt, and to get there I had to have special authorization from the French embassy, as the Prussians were approaching Würtzburg, and it was very difficult to enter. I wanted my "Blind Emperor" so much that I would have gone to the embassy that very evening if I had not been afraid to find M. de Trevise asleep.

Of all the city's museums, only M. de Sieboldt's remained open. As a Dutch officer decorated with a Prussian eagle, the colonel thought that with him present no one would dare touch his collection; while awaiting the arrival of the Prussians, all he did was walk, in his grand costume, through the three long rooms that the king had given him in the garden of the court, a kind of *palais royal*, greener and sadder than ours, surrounded by cloistered walls painted with frescoes.

In this great gloomy palace, its curiosities displayed, labeled to constitute a museum, this melancholy assemblage of objects that came from far away, wrenched from their proper milieu, Old Sieboldt seemed to be a part of it all. I came to see him every day, and we passed long hours perusing the Japanese manuscripts adorned with wooden boards, these books of science, of history, some so enormous that one had to place them on the floor in order to open them, others only as high as a finger nail, readable only with a magnifying glass, full of gold, fine and precious. M. de Sieboldt made me admire his twenty-two volume Japanese encyclopedia, or he would translate an ode from the *Hiaknin*, a marvelous work published under the supervision of the Japanese emperors, and where one finds lives, portraits, and lyric fragments of the most famous poets of the empire. Then we arranged his collection of arms, the golden helmets with large chinpieces, the breastplates, the coats of arms, and the great sabers for two hands which recall the Knight of the Temple, and with which one can so well open one's stomach.

He explained to me the love emblems painted on the gold shells, introduced me to Japanese interiors by showing me a model of his house at Edo, a miniature in lacquer representing everything, from the silk window blinds to the garden rocks, a Lilliputian garden, decorated with delicate plants of indigenous flora. What interested me very much, also, were Japanese religious objects, the little gods made of painted wood, the sacred vases, the vestments, and the portable chapels, real Pupazzi theaters, that every believer kept in a corner of his house. The small red idols are ranged in the rear, a thin knotted cord hanging on the front. Before beginning his prayer, the Japanese kneels and strikes a bell at the bottom of the altar with the cord, thus getting the attention of his gods. I was like a child in this sonorous wave, to the very ends of these Asias of the Orient where the rising sun seems all golden, from the blades of their great sabers to the edges of their small books. . . .

When I left, my eyes full of all the reflections of lacquer, jade, of brilliant colored maps, above all of the days when the colonel had read me one of the Japanese odes, a poetry so chaste, distinguished, original, so profound, the streets of Munich had a remarkable effect on me. Japan, Bavaria—two countries new to me, that I learned about at the same time, where I saw the one through the other—were confused in my mind, became a kind of vague country, a blue country. . . .

Ten days in Munich and still no news of my Japanese tragedy. I began to lose hope when, one evening, in the cafe where we took our meals, I saw our colonel arriving with a beaming face. "I have it!" he said; "come to the museum tomorrow morning. . . . We will read it together; you will see how beautiful it is." He was very animated that evening. His eyes shone when he spoke. He declaimed, out loud, passages from the tragedy and tried to sing the choruses. Two or three times his niece felt obliged to quiet him: "Ouncle, . . . ouncle. . . ." I attributed this fever and exaltation to pure lyric enthusiasm. In reality, the fragments that he recited to me seemed very beautiful, and I was impatient to possess my masterpiece.

The next day, when I arrived in the garden of the court, I was very surprised to find the collection rooms closed. The colonel's absence from his museum was so extraordinary that I ran to his house with a vague feeling of anxiety. The street he lived on, a short, calm, suburban street with gardens and low houses, seemed more animated than usual. Groups of people were talking in front of the doors. The door to the Sieboldt house was closed, the blinds open.

People entered and left looking sad. One felt there a catastrophe too large to be held within, spilling out onto the street. . . . When I arrived, I heard sobs. It was at the end of a small hallway, in a crowded light room, like a study. It had a long table in white wood, books, manuscripts, cases filled with collections, albums covered in brocaded silk, on the wall Japanese arms, prints, large maps, and in the midst of this disorder of trips and study, the colonel stretched out on his bed, his long white beard straight on his chest, with his poor little "ouncle" on her knees in a corner, crying. M. de Sieboldt had died suddenly in the night.

I left Munich that very evening, not having the courage to trouble all this sadness for a literary fantasy, and that is why I have known only the title of the marvelous Japanese tragedy "The Blind Emperor"! [Translated from Daudet, pp. 312–35.]

Philipp Franz Balthasar von Siebold was buried with the full military honors of the Bavarian court in the Old South Cemetery, Sudfriedhof, in the shadow of St. Stephan's Kirche on Thalkircher Strasse in Munich. In the same cemetery is the grave of his foster-father and teacher at Würzburg, Ignaz Döllinger. At the gate there is a list of famous men whose remains lie in the four-century-old burial ground: Pettenkoffer, the father of German hygiene; von Liebig, the chemist; and von Döllinger, the great Catholic conservative theologian and son of Siebold's former professor. Siebold is not listed as one of the distinguished persons buried in the graveyard.

The death of Philipp Siebold ended the long line of eminent medical scholars from that family. Alexander moved from his post as interpreter at the British legation to Japanese government service and became successful as a career secretary to the Japanese cabinet. He participated in official missions to London, Frankfurt, and Vienna in 1911, and his collection from Japan was deposited in a museum in the Austrian capital. In his autobiography Alexander refers to his father as an example of a Dutch factory doctor who assisted in the advance of medicine, surgery, and the natural sciences in Japan. There was a second son, Heinrich (1852–1908), and two daughters: Helene, Freifrau von Ulm Erbach; and Mathilde, Freifrau von Brandenstein. Mathilde's husband, Graf Alexander Brandenstein-Zeppelin, was a scion of the family that was destined to pioneer in German aeronautics. Their grandson, Graf Alexander von Brandenstein-Zeppelin, holds the archives of his great-grandfather, Philipp Franz von Siebold, at his castle in Mittelbiberach in Swabia.

Today there is no living heir who continues the family name of Philipp Franz von Siebold.

Siebold's accomplishments have received the greatest recognition in the country that he loved, Japan. Every Japanese school child knows the name Shīboruto as the great foreign teacher who came to their country during the fading years of the Tokugawa shogunate. In the museum hall of the Nagasaki Prefectural Library, his military uniform, his medical and surgical kit, including an obstetrical forceps, letters to Ine, and many volumes of evidence in the "Case of the Stolen Maps" are exhibited. At Narutaki, one inscription at the gate reads: "the house of Siebold *sensei*." Another reads: "Siebold is the one who deserves the glory of the great achievement to have introduced knowledge to the Japan of today." The outlines of his home are preserved through marker stones, and Japanese women come to harvest the medicinal plants that Siebold began to cultivate there almost a century and a half ago. A commanding bust of Siebold dominates the scene.

The tomb in Munich seems typical of Siebold: surrounded by classical German tombstones, his is Japanese. It is a replica of the spire of concentric tapering circles which crowns Japanese shrines and temples. On one face is inscribed: "*Philip Fr. von Siebold, Oberlt. u. Botaniker 1790–1866.*" One line on the other face reads: "*Erforscher Japans,*" explorer of Japan. Beneath are four Japanese characters, and these are the most fitting memorial for the man who was responsible for the flow of such a diversified body of knowledge between Japan and the West—they read: "such a strong bridge." No man in history has been such a remarkable bridge of knowledge that spanned the thousands of miles separating Europe and Japan.

六

CHAPTER

VI

J. L. C. Pompe van Meerdervoort:
The Official Adoption of Western Medicine

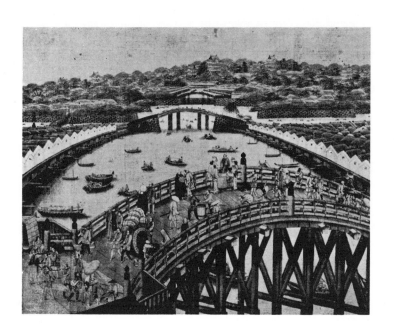

THE UNSUNG HERO of the development of Western medicine in Japan was a young and untested Dutch doctor, Johannes Lydius Catherinus Pompe van Meerdervoort. He was twenty-nine years old when he came to Nagasaki to teach medicine. His running mate was a twenty-five-year-old Japanese physician, Matsumoto Ryōjun. Neither had taught medicine, but their youthful vigor and their teamwork were essential factors in the establishment of a full-fledged medical school against odds that would have turned aside older and experienced teachers. Pompe and Matsumoto led the first successful program of international cooperation in medical education.

The shogunate recognized the pitiful state of the nation's defenses after the Perry expedition and turned to old friends, the Dutch, for support in the development of a navy. In 1855 the Japanese forwarded a request to The Hague for assistance in the establishment of a naval military school. The Hollanders were eager to strengthen their ties with Japan, and a detachment of naval officers and a frigate, the *Soembing*, a gift of the Dutch government, were ordered to Nagasaki. One year later the Japanese requested a second frigate and, in addition, the services of a Dutch naval surgeon to teach at the naval school. The leader of the new mission, W. J. C. Ridder Huyssen van Kattendyke, selected Pompe van Meerdervoort for the assignment as the naval surgeon—and it was a brilliant choice.

J. L. C. Pompe van Meerdervoort was born in Brugge on May 5, 1829, the son of a Dutch army officer. This was just one year before the separation of Belgium, which included Brugge, from The Netherlands.

Pompe entered the study of medicine at the military medical school in Utrecht in 1846. The edifice that housed the school dated back to 1348 and the Crusades. After their return from the Third Crusade, the Knights of the German Order established at Utrecht the German House, which included a monastery, church, and hospital. All of the facilities of the German House were converted to a miltiary hospital by Napoleon in 1807. After the restoration of their freedom the Dutch established military medical schools in 1815 at Leiden and Louvain. In 1822 the schools were merged and moved to the military hospital in the historic German House at Utrecht. Here the military continued to offer a three-year educational program for future medical officers until 1868. After that year, all students aspiring to careers as military medical officers entered the regular medical curriculum at Amsterdam, and, in 1881, all special programs for the education of military medical officers were terminated.

On August 16, 1849, Pompe completed his studies and received the commission of "army surgeon, third class, for marine duty." His service record shows that he was posted to the Dutch East Indies on the *Merapi* in March, 1851, and that he served in Sumatra during a native uprising, in the Moluccas for a leprosy survey, and in New Guinea. Pompe returned to Holland in the summer of 1855 and one year later, in August, 1856, was successful in the examination for promotion to the rank of army surgeon, second class. The next entry in his service record, February 1, 1857, was for an assignment to the "propeller ship *Japan*" and passage to the Dutch East Indies.*

The *Japan* arrived at Nagasaki on September 22, 1857. Shortly after, Pompe was, in his words, "informed by The Netherlands commissioner that the Japanese government had expressed a wish to have some of their own medical students instructed in the medical and surgical sciences, and that the arrangements should be as I pleased" (Pompe van Meerdervoort, 1859, p. 211). Pompe was told that this request was based on the full acceptance by the shogunate of the fact that Dutch medicine was superior to the indigenous system.

It is clear that Pompe came to Japan unaware that he was destined to be the founder of a medical school. He carried none of the essentials of a teaching program—no textbooks, laboratory manuals, charts, or specimens for demonstration. When he reached Deshima he found a few texts in the surgeon's quarters, including a Dutch translation of *Die Cellularpathologie in ihrer Begrundung auf physiologische und pathologische Gewebelehre* by

* The *Japan*, a frigate of three hundred tons, was purchased by the Japanese government and renamed the *Kanrin Maru*. In 1860 it sailed from Yokohama to San Francisco as escort to the U.S.S. *Powhatan*, bearing a delegation of Japanese to ratify the Treaty of Amity and Commerce between Japan and the United States.

Virchow. With such a complete lack of teaching aids, Pompe could easily have settled for a few lectures in natural history and therapeutics. But he was determined from the beginning to establish a complete five-year program in medical education beginning with the premedical sciences.

Shortly after Pompe's arrival, the international style of the school was set when he was joined by a gifted and attractive young physician from the shogunate at Edo, Matsumoto Ryōjun. A court physician, Matsumoto was a practitioner of *Kampō* but had also studied Western medicine with his distinguished physician-father, Satō Taizen. When Matsumoto married, his father-in-law had no male heir and followed the Japanese tradition of adopting Matsumoto and anointing him with the family name to assure the family succession.

When Matsumoto Ryōjun learned of the impending establishment of a program to teach Western medicine at Nagasaki, he requested permission from the shogunate to study with Pompe and to assist in the development of the new school. This request, however, posed a difficult problem for the authority. In 1849, under pressure from Confucian reactionaries, the shogunate had forbidden the study of Western medicine. Therefore, it could hardly give official sanction for one of the court physicians to study Western medicine at Nagasaki. However, convinced of the importance of Western medicine, the *bakufu* sent Matsumoto to Nagasaki in disguise. He was designated officially as a student at the naval school with the full knowledge that he would study Western medicine. From the first day of their acquaintance, Pompe found Matsumoto a person who commanded respect. "I met him and discovered that he was a person with a sound knowledge" (translated from Pompe van Meerdervoort, 1867–68, p. 179). This was the beginning of a remarkable relationship—Pompe, the leader, but dependent for success on Matsumoto, who was always his dedicated and able second lieutenant. The bans against the study of Western medicine were easily evaded by having the medical students formally enrolled in the naval school.

Matsumoto assumed the responsibility for the selection of the students, and the first class, numbering twelve in all, included students from the court at Edo and from five of the feudatories on Kyūshū. Several of the students who had been practitioners of *Kampō* were over forty years of age and, eager to resume their practices, asked Matsumoto to arrange a shorter curriculum. However, Pompe would have nothing but the best and refused to offer any program in medicine other than the full five-year educational sequence.

Instead of using a small, dark room behind the palisades of Deshima where Kaempfer, Thunberg, and Siebold had held their classes in medicine, Pompe presented his first lecture in the heart of Nagasaki—in a building belonging to the Japanese government. November 15, 1857, was a memorable day, for it marked Pompe's first effort as a teacher. He discussed the influences of the natural sciences on civilization and their importance in the study of medicine and surgery. At the end of the lecture his enthusiasm for his task in Japan was heightened by a singular ceremony: "the senior student, or rather the one highest in rank among them, in behalf of himself and the others thanked me in a few hearty words for the kindness shown in entering their mission and in now commencing my new task as their instructor, assuring me that they had long felt the want of greater facilities and aids in scientific pursuits, which hitherto had been much retarded by their old institutions and system of government" (1859, p. 212). For any teacher such words would have been gratifying, but for Pompe, after his first lecture to any class and in a foreign land, they were singularly heart-warming. The candor of the students in admitting their own deficiencies made him more determined than ever to develop a model program.

When he met the students on the following day, Pompe learned that teaching methods at Utrecht could not be applied in Japan. He was eager to know how much of his first lecture had gotten through to the students and as well to appraise their background knowledge in the natural sciences. But when he asked the students to respond to his questions orally, they were embarrassed. Their embarrassment became acute when they were unable to answer many of Pompe's questions before their classmates, the interpreters, and Matsumoto.

One of Matsumoto's most important contributions throughout the five years of their association was his role as the medium for

179

communication between Pompe and the students. Pompe knew no Japanese, and only a few of the students knew even a smattering of Dutch. A complicated sequence was developed. Pompe lectured in Dutch; Nagasaki interpreters stood beside him and translated the lecture into Japanese, and Matsumoto with brush and rice paper transcribed the lectures in Japanese for subsequent distribution to the students.

As the program developed, Pompe recognized that the Nagasaki interpreters were unfamiliar with medical terminology and that their translations were often inaccurate. With characteristic thoroughness Pompe took several steps to improve communications. He began an intensive study of Japanese and in time was able to detect at least some of the inaccuracies in the translations of his lectures. He also prepared detailed outlines of his lectures which were translated into Japanese by Matsumoto and distributed to the students before the lectures. A third step was the initiation of classes in Dutch by a teacher from the naval school who was a Hollander.

Yet, despite these efforts, Pompe continued to rely on Matsumoto and the interpreters. The almost insurmountable difficulties posed by the lack of a common language were described by a student, Nagayo Sensai, who had joined Pompe's class at the recommendation of Nagayo's former teacher, Ogata Kōan. He attended his first lecture in January, 1860: "Dr. Matsumoto introduced me to Dr. Pompe, but I could not speak a word and just shook hands, because he was the first foreigner I ever saw. When the lecture began, the subject was on general pathology and was interpreted by Nishi Keitarō. I could not understand a word-by-word translation. I was just struck with surprise. However, only Matsumoto Ryōjun and Shiba Ryōkai could understand his speech and were always taking notes" (translated from Nagayo, p. 11).

Two and a half years after the first class, in the spring of 1860, Bishop George Smith from Victoria, Hong Kong, was an interested visitor to Pompe's classroom:

> . . . the name of each disease was written on a blackboard in European characters and in the Latin language. Dr. Pompe delivered his lecture partly extempore and partly from a manu-

script in the Dutch language. A Japanese interpreter rendered it into the native colloquial language, which was rapidly committed to writing by a Japanese reporter. The manuscript of the latter formed a text-book for the native students, who were thus enabled to pursue their studies afterwards at leisure and in detail. This copyist (Matsumoto Ryōjun) was assistant to the lecturer, and was destined to be the medical officer in the Siogoon's palace [Smith, p. 219].

The five-year curriculum that Pompe projected followed the Dutch pattern. The students began their studies with the premedical subjects—physics, chemistry, and biology. These were followed by instruction in anatomy, histology, physiology, pathology, pharmacology and therapeutics, general medicine, surgery, and ophthalmology. Pompe soon recognized that the students were especially attracted to exercises in which they could utilize their manual dexterity and introduced instruction and practice in bandaging with the premedical sciences. When he began to lecture on pharmacology, Nagasaki practitioners who were anxious to learn the details of compounding Western prescriptions joined the medical students.

Pompe acceded to a request that he teach mineralogy, and this extended his lecture schedule to include two evenings a week; the preparation of these lectures was facilitated by the many new European texts on natural science, mining, geology, and mineralogy that he found at Nagasaki. The mineralogy students brought samples of minerals which Pompe collected for the Rijksmuseum at Leiden.

The number of students rose rapidly. Just seven months after the opening of the school there were twenty-three studying medicine and surgery and twenty who were concentrating on the natural sciences—physics, chemistry, geology, and mineralogy. Their dedication to learning was Pompe's greatest satisfaction. In the physics classes the ambition of the students was "unbounded. Seldom do I see any one of them who is not all attention" (Pompe van Meerdervoort, 1859, p. 213). The students from the feudatories were more zealous than the self-assured students from the shogun's court. If the students did not understand a discussion in the lecture, on the following day

181

they politely submitted a written request to Pompe for further explanation.

A singular accolade came from Ogata Kōan when he enrolled his son as a student with Pompe and Matsumoto. Ogata wrote to a friend, Takeya Ryōtei: "I heard that Pompe, Siebold, and others have been very active in Nagasaki and I am thinking about sending my son there. I appreciate your comment that the manners of students there are bad. But it would be profitable for my son to get into close contact with Westerners, and I am planning to send my first son, Heizō, there" (translated from Numata, 1966, p. 19). Ogata Heizō enrolled as a student at Pompe's school in the autumn of 1859.

Pompe's respect for Matsumoto mounted steadily: "To a clever judgment he joins an unlimited ambition for all science, he has a strong and decisive character, and he is always ready to sacrifice his comfort and his life to alleviate the sufferings of humankind" (translated from Pompe van Meerdervoort, 1867–68, p. 221).

Just seven months after his arrival, Pompe joined a memorable expedition to visit several of the Kyūshū *daimyō* who had repeatedly invited the Hollanders to their feudatories. They sailed on the *Japan* with Japanese officers and crew; there were also Dutch naval officers aboard as navigational advisers. When they reached Shimonoseki, they spent the night in the *ryokan* that had been used for two centuries by the Dutch captains and their embassies on the *hofreis* to Edo. Pompe was especially interested in the images of his Dutch predecessors which had been carved on the doors and posts of the *ryokan* by Japanese artists. When they reached Kagoshima they were impressed by the impact of Western technology: a small steamship, blast furnaces, excavators, glassworks, and artillery had been developed.

In the autumn of 1859 Pompe made a similar cruise to Hakata in northwest Kyūshū and treated a distinguished *daimyō*, Kuroda Narihiro. Fortunately, Kuroda, lord of the Fukuoka clan, described his contact with Pompe in detail in a letter to a friend, Date Munenari, lord of the Uwajima clan:

The two government steamships, making the navigation training, arrived at Hakata on the 18th. Kimura Tosho, trainees, and some

Dutchmen were on board the royal ship *Edo*. Katsu Rintarō, trainees, some Dutchmen, and some students of various clans were on board the royal ship *Nippon*. Kimura and all other members wanted to meet me and he asked me whether they could meet me and I could visit the ship. I asked to be excused from the invitation because I had been sick in bed due to lumbago. Kimura Hajime came again and said that I would better be examined by Pompe, who fortunately was on board the ship, and that the Dutchmen were worrying very much about my health and wondering whether I could go to Hakozaki by a palanquin and meet Pompe there. I asked to be excused from this again. Then Kimura said that Pompe was willing even to come to the castle, since the visit of foreigners to the castle had not been rare. My chief retainers were concerned about these matters because I had recently asked the shogunate to postpone my attendance at the government office. Kimura said that he and Katsu would assure that I need not worry about the shogunate, since I was going to see Pompe because of my illness.

Thus I went to Hakozaki and met Pompe. He examined me and gave detailed instructions on medication to Ryōtei (Kuroda's physician named Takeya Ryōtei). He recommended the use of potassium iodide, cod-liver oil, and massage. Ryōtei said that iodide was available in Hakata, but he could not get cod-liver oil. Pompe was kind enough to offer the cod-liver oil to me. It would be rather difficult for me to recover completely from rheumatism, but he told me that these special drugs would be beneficial in my illness.

Ryōtei talked with Pompe about various subjects, and he learned a lot from Pompe. I also had many questions to ask him, but we talked only for a while, since I did not feel well. I met Matsumoto Ryōjun, Pompe's first student, and I thought he would be an excellent physician. I regret that I have not written in detail, since I have been occupied with many other things. Pompe told us that photography was so difficult to use that he had never used it and that it required a skill in Holland.

Although I did not see them, the Dutchmen were very good at horse riding. . . . I was relieved to see that their visit went on very smoothly. Originally they were planning to sail from here to Uwajima, but they returned from here to Nagasaki this time. I want you to know that they will probably sail to your country next year, although I am not sure. It may be convenient for you if they will visit you after your return to your castle from Edo [translated from Numata, 1966, p. 39].

Pompe considered anatomy to be the linchpin for his program, but it was his major frustration for two years. The Nagasaki officials would not comply with Pompe's repeated requests for a cadaver for his classes in anatomy. He relied on lectures and a few charts prepared at Nagasaki: "the officers of the government fear to give their consent to it as it conflicts with the moral and religious institutions of the Japanese people. . . . My instruction has been by demonstrations on engravings, but every anatomist will agree with me that this is a very unsatisfactory way to teach anatomy" (Pompe van Meerdervoort, 1859, pp. 218–19). Another factor that mitigated against Pompe was that he was a foreigner and a Christian, and the voices of the Confucian reactionaries were influential in the land. On several occasions Matsumoto requested authorization for human corpses, but he too was unsuccessful.

A few of Pompe's students who were traditionalists expressed a preference for study from engravings rather than from a human body, but the majority shared Pompe's zeal—and his frustration. In addition to the engravings, Pompe dissected the heads and eyes of cows for the students, and after one year a papier-mâché model of a human body arrived from France. Such models were used widely at that time in European anatomical theaters and the most accurate were those manufactured in Paris.

After almost two years Pompe's requests for a cadaver were finally heeded on September 3, 1859. Several of his students reported to him with great secrecy and equal delight that the governor of Nagasaki had just received orders from Edo to turn over a corpse for dissection. Of immediate significance was the fact that an execution was to take place within six days.

The elaborate preparations to avoid public demonstrations consumed all of the time and effort of Pompe, his associates, and the Nagasaki officials. The government could not permit a permanent building to be defiled by a post-mortem examination. Therefore, a temporary shed was hastily thrown together which Pompe agreed to destroy as soon as the dissection had been completed. The site of the shed was beside the execution ground where more than two and a half centuries earlier, in 1597, twenty-six Christians, including a physician-priest, had been martyred. The isolated location on this rocky promontory was a further sign of the deep anxiety of the Nagasaki officials that there would be assaults by citizens incensed at the violation of a cultural attitude which had endured for many centuries. Pompe's pupils were also apprehensive that the people would riot to prevent the autopsy.

Despite the strong public antagonism that was believed to prevail (and the secrecy with which the plans for the dissection had been shrouded), there were many requests from physicians and laymen for permission to attend the now widely heralded event. A skilled craftsman of cutlery was the only layman permitted to attend. Pompe hoped that such an experience would improve the man's proficiency to a degree that Japan would become self-sufficient in the manufacture of surgical instruments.

After two years of frustration it is not surprising that Pompe painted a detailed and vivid picture of a memorable event in Japanese medicine. As another move to thwart public hostility and to facilitate transfer of the corpse to the dissection shed, the execution was performed in the inner court of the prison instead of on the public execution ground. The criminal was an old hand at robbery and this was his third offense. Other crimes for which capital punishment was always the penalty included regicide, patricide, incendiarism, and the murder of one's teacher.

The executioner was, in Pompe's opinion, a master hand, for the single wound which severed the spinous process of the sixth cervical vertebra showed that the head, which was brought to Pompe separately in a basket, had been cut off at one stroke. The actual beheading followed a prescribed procedure:

> The criminal is placed on his knees, while the hands are placed with the palms uppermost, but he is not blindfolded. A foot and a half before the place where the man is kneeling, they make a hole in the ground, several feet long, broad, and deep. The executioner is at the left side, and an assistant, also in a kneeling position, is on the left side. The latter takes the right foot in his hand and makes three signals behind the criminal's back. At the third signal the head is cut off and falls into the hole. At the same moment the assistant lifts up the right extremity with some force so that the body falls forward and the bleeding neck comes just above the hole [1860, p. 88].

185

Twenty-one medical students and twenty-four physicians attended the dissection which began on September 9 and continued for two days. This was probably the first scientific dissection in Japan. Pompe dissected one arm and allowed the students to dissect the other. After six hours Pompe turned to his other duties, but the students were so enthusiastic that they continued until dark with only a fifteen-minute interval for dinner. And when darkness fell they marched to the residence of the governor and obtained his official permission to continue the dissection for a second day. After the dissection was completed, Buddhist priests carried away the corpse and burned it in their traditional funeral ritual.

A second body was turned over to Pompe two months later, on November 7, 1859, and this dissection was attended by sixty students and physicians: "what is most remarkable, *one Japanese lady* was also present! She is an accoucheuse, who has studied the medical science, and she earnestly requested me to permit her to witness the dissection, which I allowed, and I must say that she neglected nothing. She always was very attentive and asked me several questions which proved her to be very intelligent; she assisted also in the operations" (*ibid.*, p. 91). The lady was of distinguished lineage: she was Ine, the daughter of Philipp Siebold.

In the summer of 1858 Pompe had a singular opportunity to demonstrate the importance of Western medicine: "In July, 1858, the American warship *Mississippi* brought us cholera from China" (translated from Pompe van Meerdervoort, 1867–68, p. 169). (The records of the Navy Department in Washington do not show any evidence of cholera on the battleship. A description of the cruise by one of the officers reports an outbreak of diarrhea on departure from China, but there is nothing to suggest that this was a disease of the severity of cholera. There were, however, many Chinese hulls that sailed between Shanghai and Nagasaki without the health regulations required on an American man-of-war.)

Unfortunately, the epidemic was a severe one. It spread rapidly from Nagasaki across the empire and there were 12,000 deaths in

Edo in the month of August. With little faith in their physicians, the people turned to the priests:

> The monotonous sounds of a Buddhist chaunt and beating of a hollow piece of wood, are frequently heard from the interior of a Japanese dwelling, in which some inmate of the household lies prostrate with fever or is afflicted with any other of the prevalent forms of sickness. The priests employed belong to various classes of sacerdotal rank and wear different styles of vestment, from the coarse garb of the priestly servitor and acolyte to the prelatic robe of the abbot of the temple. Many of the priests are boys serving apprenticeship to some elder priest, engaged partly in the menial duties of the temple. Buddhist nuns too are not uncommon of all ages, from the young girl of tender years to the decrepit and septuagenarian priestess.
>
> In the houses of the sick, boy-priests are often seen engaged in their superstitious rites for expelling the evil demons which bring calamity and for propitiating the favourable influence of their divinities. Charms and incantations performed by the priesthood are supposed to have their meritorious power; and the Bonzes are in greater request than the physicians. On one occasion observing a sick man surrounded by the noisy clatter of Buddhist sound-boards and bells accompanying the monotonous prayer of the priest, we learnt on inquiry that the friends of the sufferer had not yet sent for medical help. On other occasions we discovered proofs of the popular mind in such cases being more impressed with the supernatural than with the physical remedies within their reach. A priest's gratuity is more willingly paid than a doctor's fee [Smith, pp. 92–93].

As the outbreak in Nagasaki began to wane, Pompe prepared a short monograph describing his therapy. He recommended the use of Peruvian bark for fever, and opium followed by hot baths for the violent intestinal cramps. In this regime he was following a program developed by K. R. A. Wunderlich, professor of medicine at Leipzig, based on Wunderlich's experience in several major waves of cholera that developed in Europe after 1860. The monograph was translated into Japanese by Matsumoto and circulated widely in Japan. Matsumoto sent a copy of Pompe's monograph to Ogata Kōan, who recommended alternative programs. On the basis of Pompe's monograph and information from several European texts, Ogata prepared a monograph, *Korera Chijun* [Standard therapy for cholera].

187

The drama of Pompe van Meerdervoort's role in the cholera epidemic was described in a letter from Kuroda Narihiro, the lord of the Fukuoka clan, to Date Muneshiro, lord of the Uwajima clan:

> A sort of communicable disease is rampant in Nagasaki these days. Scores are dying every day. At the maximum, sixty patients died in one day. The magistrate inquired of the Dutch physician [Pompe] about the disease and he was told that this was cholera. He asked the Dutchman to treat patients, and found that many people recovered. On the other hand, all of the patients died who were treated by the physicians of the Chinese school. Even people who do not like Hollanders have started to ask for his help. I received what the Dutchman mentioned as to the precautions on daily food and drink during the epidemic and the way of treatment. Since it is possible that this epidemic may reach Edo, I explained recently to Tozuka Seikai what I have heard. Please ask Seikai about details. I have just received the written statement of the Dutchman, and made several copies of it, which are already distributed [translated from Numata, 1966, p. 22].

And by another physician: "Thank you very much for your copy of Pompe's booklet written at the time of the cholera outbreak in Nagasaki. As Pompe predicted, the outbreak also started in the city [Edo], being rampant in the Tsukiji Hatchōbori and Akasaka areas at the beginning" (*ibid.*, p. 24). Pompe himself contracted a mild form of the disease but was back at work in thirteen days.

From the time of his arrival in Nagasaki, Pompe crusaded for the establishment of a teaching hospital. He emphasized its importance not only for the medical school and the general welfare of the citizens of Nagasaki but also as a resource for the crews of the increasing number of foreign vessels that were entering Nagasaki.

In June, 1858, eight months after the opening of the medical school, Pompe prepared a detailed memorandum on the design of a hospital which Donker Curtius, the *opperhoofd* and consul for the Dutch, presented to the shogunate. A copy of this memorandum has been preserved in the archives of the Shimazu family, and Professor Numata Jirō has reproduced it in his detailed and valuable study of Pompe. Pompe placed great emphasis on the importance of fresh air. He stated that the building should be on a hilltop and should be "H" shaped with the opening of the "H" toward the prevailing winds. He recommended that a large window be cut in the ceiling; that all windows be kept open twelve months a year; that no trees should be planted on the grounds, because they might impede the flow of fresh air. As a further emphasis on sanitation, Pompe recommended that special attention should be paid to water supply by choosing a site beside a clear, running stream. "A swamp with stagnant water should be avoided. The hospital should always have enough supply of clear water of good quality, since its water consumption is great" (*ibid.*, p. 29). Eight fifteen-bed wards should be used to segregate patients with specific diseases: febrile diseases, skin diseases, syphilis, trauma, internal diseases, eye diseases, scabies, and the eighth ward for convalescent patients. He also recommended that one room should be set aside as a library.

Pompe received strong support from the Nagasaki magistrate, Okabe Suruga, who with Nagai Genba presented a formal endorsement for the plan to the shogunate. Matsumoto Ryōjun also urged the government to make the necessary funds available. Despite the endorsements of Nagasaki officials, more than two years passed before authorization was received. Pompe attributed this delay to the reluctance of the Japanese to have a foreigner supervise a government-supported program.

Pompe's untiring efforts during the cholera epidemic were a major factor in the favorable decision finally reached by the shogunate. He supervised the construction of the hospital Yōjōsho, and the plans were exactly along the lines that he had recommended. The shogunate gave him responsibility for every aspect of the development except the regulations concerned with the selection of patients. They wished to reserve admissions to the upper classes. Pompe, however, was adamant that he must be responsible for admissions policies and his insistence prevailed. The hospital with one hundred and twenty beds was opened for patients on September 21, 1861, four years after Pompe's arrival in Japan. Adjoining Yōjōsho was a new medical-school building which included a lecture hall, demonstration room, and dormitories.

The regulations governing admission and care in the hospital were explicit:

1. A person who wishes to be treated should come directly to the hospital, being accompanied by a guarantor. He should bring duplicate applications with the signatures of the village officer and guarantor; one should be presented at the gate office, and another at the main entrance. He will be admitted after the inquiry of officers and physicians. Since the hospital will inquire into the identity of the patient, it is suggested that he report to the village chief before coming to the hospital. However, the hospital can admit a patient without the request of the village chief.

2. The hospital will furnish bedding. If a patient wishes to bring his own, he may be allowed to use it after the physician's inspection.

3. A convalescent patient who is able to walk may return home, even though he is still on medication. However, he should visit the hospital regularly for treatment thereafter.

4. A person from a well-established family should pay six *monmes* a day to cover all the expenses during hospitalization. He may pay before or after recovery, depending upon his convenience.

5. A person who wishes to bring his own attendant to the hospital and occupy a single room should pay twelve *monmes* a day.

6. Free medication will be given to a person who is not well financed, so that he should pay one *monme* and five *bus* a day. If he is very poor, he may be excused from all payment, depending upon the circumstance.

7. The patient's relatives and other visitors should bring the numbered card which has been given beforehand, and must meet the patient accompanied by a hospital guide. If they wish to bring food as a present, it must be inspected by the physician [*ibid.*].

Several weeks after the opening of Yōjōsho, seventy patients had been admitted. In the febrile disease ward there were cases of typhoid fever, cholera, and smallpox; the venereal disease ward was crowded. Sailors from the many foreign ships in Nagasaki harbor were admitted with fractures and other forms of trauma. The clinic was filled with patients suffering primarily from tuberculosis, heart diseases, skin diseases, eye diseases, and venereal disease.

The opening of the hospital added another major responsibility to Pompe's back-breaking schedule, but he liked it. He climbed the hill from Deshima to Yōjōsho each morning, arriving at eight o'clock to start his rounds in the hospital. Each student was assigned a task for the morning; some cleaned and bandaged ulcers and other skin infections; others were set to work on the patients' charts; while a third group was assigned to the pharmacy to compound prescriptions. Pompe did not hesitate to be strict and demanding with the students in his constant striving for excellence.

After the morning's rounds he lectured for two hours and taught materia medica in the hospital pharmacy. There was a second two-hour lecture at three o'clock, after which he made evening rounds, attended patients in the clinic, and, as dusk approached, left the hospital to visit patients in their homes accompanied by Matsumoto as the interpreter and several students.

The number of practicing physicians who attended his lectures mounted steadily. They appeared in traditional robes carrying a single sword and with head shaved in the style of a Buddhist priest. Each physician was followed by a servant bearing on his back a portable dispensary. Occasionally an unlicensed practitioner appeared with head unshaven and no sword. The unlicensed practitioners ranked far down in the social order, with apothecaries and other artisans, beneath the farmers.

It was not long before Pompe became aware of the fact that the hospital beds were monopolized by government officers and people of the higher classes. Despite the hospital regulation of welcoming patients from all strata of society, there were no artisans, farmers, or merchants in the clinics or wards:

> I soon noticed that many Japanese visiting the hospital were relatively wealthy, and many were government officers. The public regarded the hospital as a special institution for the privileged classes or a shelter for government officers. It is characteristic of the nation that laborers did not want to be treated in the same way as higher classes, and they did not wish to be admitted to the hospital. Even if they had wanted to come to the hospital, they would have been rejected by their village officers. As soon as I confirmed these facts, I tried to do all I

could to cope with this social system. A hospital should be for all people. I did not object to treating wealthy people also, but they should not be treated at the sacrifice of poor people [translated from Pompe van Meerdervoort, 1867–68, p. 214].

Pompe renewed his insistence with the Japanese authorities that all citizens must be admitted and finally was victorious.

A painful cross that Pompe van Meerdervoort bore during his five years in Japan was to see at first hand the deteriorating position of his country in Japan. The vicissitudes of life at Deshima had been borne by the Dutch for more than two centuries with the anticipation that when Japan was opened to the West the Hollanders would be the favored nation. It was a cruel blow to see the embassies from the United States, Britain, and France rise to dominance after the many years of exclusively Dutch relationships. Nagasaki was now isolated from the main thrust of foreign influence which was occurring in Edo. Pompe felt that his heroic achievements had not received the recognition that they deserved. His frustrations were made greater by the fact that he was approaching mental and physical exhaustion.

Pompe requested orders to return to Holland in 1862 and his successor, Dr. Antonius F. Bauduin, arrived at Nagasaki in September of that year. The following month Pompe awarded diplomas to sixty-one students. He graded twenty-two of them as excellent, sixteen as good, and twenty-three as fair. One hundred and fifty students had studied medicine or natural history with Pompe at Nagasaki.

On November 1, 1862, just over five years after his arrival in Japan, Pompe van Meerdervoort sailed for Holland accompanied by two medical students, Itō Hosei and Hayashi Kenkai, five military naval students, and two civilian students who would continue their studies in The Netherlands.

A number of Pompe's students achieved distinction in medicine in Japan. Hashimoto Tsunatsune was the founder of the Red Cross hospital system which covered Japan with the most extensive national medical program before World War II.

There could have been no greater change for Pompe than to move from the exciting life at Nagasaki to the practice of general medicine in the tranquility of The Hague. He served as the physician and counselor for Japanese citizens who came to Holland, ranging from the Japanese ambassador to Japanese students studying medicine, naval tactics, law, and economics.

Pompe kept a diary of his life and work in Japan and accumulated an extensive collection of Japanese books, maps, art forms, minerals, and medical materials. Tragically, all of these were lost when the vessel on which they had been shipped, the *Calypso*, sank. But he set himself the task of preparing from memory a detailed account of his work in Japan. In 1867–68 *Vijf Jaren in Japan (1857–1863)*, in two volumes, was published at Leiden. There are chapters on Japanese history and culture, the intrusions of the West, the opening of the country, and, finally, his own work at Nagasaki. By all odds the most interesting part of the book is the detailed description of the development of the medical school and the hospital at Nagasaki. Unfortunately, it has not been translated into English; a section has been translated into Japanese.

Pompe's contributions in Japan were recognized by meritorious awards: from William III, "Knight of The Netherlands Lion"; from Lisbon, "Knight of the Royal Military Order of Our Lady of Conception of Villa Vicosa"; from the czar, "Order of St. Anna"; from Japan, the "Fourth Order of Merit with Petit Cordon of the Rising Sun."

The International Red Cross was a natural outlet for Pompe's interests and he was an official delegate from Holland to the first meeting of that organization, which was held in The Hague. In 1870 he organized and led a Red Cross hospital at Saarbrucken during the Franco-Prussian War.

Heart-warming recognition came from one of Pompe's former students in 1874. Enomoto Takeaki had gone to the Court of the Czar of All the Russias as the first Japanese envoy extraordinary and minister plenipotentiary. He asked his former teacher at Nagasaki to come to St. Petersburg as his adviser, and Pompe spent two years, 1875–77, in Russia.

On September 29, 1887, twenty years and eight days after his arrival at Nagasaki, Pompe attended the International Red Cross Congress in Karlsruhe, Germany, and discussed his years in

Japan with Mori Ōgai, an assistant to the Japanese representative. Pompe expressed to Mori his great delight that the Japanese delegate had delivered a major address before the assembly. He said that he finally felt that his five years in Japan had come to full fruition: "What I did in Japan now has historical significance." But in keen memory of the past he added as an aside: "I really met with various difficulties in those days" (translated from Numata, 1966, p. 1).

Pompe van Meerdervoort died in September, 1908, at the age of eighty, at Bergen op Zoom in The Netherlands. Until his death he continued to serve as physician for the Japanese who came to Holland. His last contribution to Japanese history was to serve as the obstetrician for the wife of the Japanese consul, Ōtori, at the birth of her third son, Ranzaburō ("Dutch third son") Ōtori. Professor Extraordinary Ranzaburō Ōtori is today one of Japan's leading scholars in the history of medicine and, naturally, an authority on the life and contributions of Pompe van Meerdervoort.

Matsumoto Ryōjun was appointed director of the Institute for Western Medicine in 1863. In the fighting that attended the Meiji Restoration he was captured in the field. When peace was restored, Matsumoto was appointed the surgeon general of the new imperial army, the first man to serve in that command.

Today, when there is so much interest in international programs, the remarkable accomplishment of Pompe and Matsumoto deserves analysis. What were the secrets of their success? One was the long-standing relationship between their countries, which generated mutual respect and confidence. The time in history was propitious; the Hollanders wished to maintain their status in Japan, and the Japanese recognized an urgent need for foreign support. The importance of Western medicine was accepted by Japanese leaders, and the rulers had taken the lead in seeking an educational program from the West. But the most important factors in the success of the program were, as is always true, the men themselves; they were young, they were not fettered by any academic traditions, they respected each other, and they were dedicated to their goals. Today, who would dream of sending a totally inexperienced twenty-nine-year-old military medical

194

officer to establish a medical school in a country where he had no facility in the language—the most difficult language in the world? And would his counterpart running mate be a twenty-five-year-old physician who also had no previous experience as a teacher? Perhaps these "handicaps" made Pompe and Matsumoto so successful at Nagasaki.

The most stirring picture of the medical center at Nagasaki shows the Dutch and Japanese flags flying side by side—just as Pompe van Meerdervoort and Matsumoto Ryōjun worked hand in hand in a truly international undertaking in medicine.

The Official Adoption of Western Medicine

Pompe van Meerdervoort was the last of the great European medical pioneers to contribute to the rise of Western medicine in Japan. The development of the medical school and teaching hospital also represented the final grandeur for Nagasaki in that epoch; after Pompe all major developments emanated from Edo.

Vaccination against smallpox was introduced by a Deshima doctor, Otto Mohnike, in 1849. Nine years later, in 1858, Shutōjo ("vaccination institute") was established in Edo. This was the same year in which the first practitioners of Western internal medicine were appointed to attend the shogun.

Shutōjo was maintained by private subscriptions and by the five physicians who constituted its founding body. As a sign of the importance attached to vaccination, about eighty physicians applied for membership in the first year, and in 1859 the government began to make an annual appropriation to Shutōjō. The following year the name was changed to Seiyō Igakujo ("Institute for Western medical education"); dormitories were erected, and students were admitted for limited instruction in Western medicine.

The early directors were among the leading physicians of Japan and exemplified the importance that was attached to the institute. The first, Ōtsuki Shunsai, was succeeded in 1862 by Ogata Kōan, and the name of the school was shortened to Igakujo. The following year Matsumoto Ryōjun assumed the directorship.

195

In November, 1867, the shogun left his castle in Edo and the emperor Meiji was restored to the position of true imperial prestige. As Meiji moved his throne from Kyoto to Edo, the name Edo was discarded and Tokyo ("eastern capital") became the name for the new seat of the mikado. Leading governmental posts passed to young liberals who, continuing the spirit of the *Rangakusha*, were determined to adopt the programs of Western nations which seemed best suited to bring Japan rapidly and efficiently to a position comparable to the leading countries of the West.

The aims of the new government were set forth in an imperial proclamation, known as the Charter Oath of Five Articles, at Kyoto on April 6, 1868. The last article stated: "Wisdom and knowledge shall be sought after in all parts of the world to establish firmly the foundations of the Empire" (Yanaga, p. 107). Missions visited the United States, Britain, France, and Germany to assess governmental structure, military organization, the courts, and other systems. For medical education, however, there was no need to dispatch a mission; the German system was the overwhelming choice—and for good reason. It was by all odds the best system in the world.

As we have noted, after military defeats the king of Prussia wisely determined early in the nineteenth century to compensate for a lack of military might with achievements in intellectual might, including medicine. The decision to achieve intellectual might was fortuitous, for medicine was ready for drastic changes. In the preceding centuries new knowledge had come from practicing physicians and had been based primarily upon their observations of patients in the hospital wards and at the autopsy table. As Abraham Flexner has noted, in the nineteenth century progress came to depend upon an interaction between the laboratory and the clinic (1925). The reformed German universities offered the environment for such developments, and the medical faculties turned away from clinical and post-mortem studies to the basic sciences. Clio Medica moved from the great Paris teaching hospitals across the Rhine to Germany. In the very year that Japan declared for the West (1868), from his little attic laboratories at the École Normale, Pasteur put the case poignantly: "Rich and large laboratories have been growing in

Germany for the last thirty years and many more are still being built; at Berlin and Bonn two palaces, worth four million francs each, are being erected for chemical studies" (Vallery-Radot, p. 152).

After 1850 Germany became the mecca for students from the other countries of continental Europe, the United States, and Britain. When the Japanese made their choice, there was no question that Germany led the world in medicine.

Another factor that influenced the decision to adopt the German system was the shadow of a German whom the Japanese knew had only masqueraded as a Hollander—Philipp Franz von Siebold. They remembered him as the greatest foreign scholar in the history of the empire, and in every activity—his lectures, his relationships, and his character—he was in all respects a forceful ambassador of his fatherland.

Further evidence of the excellence of German medicine was the predominance of German medical texts in the hands of the Japanese students of medicine. These appeared in Dutch or Japanese translations, but there was little question as to their German origin.

The Reverend Guido Fridolin Verbeck, an American missionary, played an important role in the adoption of German medicine. In 1853, at the age of twenty-three, after emigrating to the United States from The Netherlands, he studied and practiced engineering but then turned to the clergy and foreign missions. He went to Nagasaki under the banner of the Dutch Reformed Church and, after studying Japanese, opened a school to teach English. He was a resourceful missionary and, since preaching Christian doctrine was forbidden, delivered his religious messages by using the New Testament as the English primer for his classes. Verbeck's school was so successful that it was officially recognized and sponsored by the *bakufu* in 1863. In 1868 Verbeck was invited to Tokyo to serve as adviser to several of his former students who had assumed important roles in the development of the outstanding Imperial University in Tokyo. He became the leading foreign adviser on educational developments for the government.

A year after Verbeck moved to Tokyo, Igakujo was designated

as the East College of the University, and the administration of both the medical school and its hospital was entrusted to two physicians, Sagara Chian and Iwasa Jun.

The question now arose as to the system of medicine that should be adopted. At this time, although the Japanese felt a lingering attachment to the Dutch, they were dedicated to adopting the programs of more powerful nations. They felt a sense of gratitude to a British missionary surgeon, Willis, who had worked heroically on the casualties in the battles of the Restoration. To settle the debt and to remove Willis from the picture, he was sent to far-off Kagoshima with an inflated salary. When Verbeck's opinion on the question was sought, he stated that there was no better medicine in the world than German medicine. Sagara Chian then became an ardent advocate of the German system and in 1870 transmitted an official request to the government that German professors be invited to teach at the medical school. He also asked that the unclaimed bodies of criminals be made available to the medical school for dissection. The Cabinet affirmed that medicine would be developed on the German pattern, and the German consul, Max August Scipio von Brandt, was asked to arrange for German professors to come to Japan. In his dispatch to Berlin, Brandt suggested that the first professors should be high-ranking military officers so that they would be readily accepted by the nobility. Leopold Mueller and Theodore Hoffmann, both Prussian military surgeons, arrived at Yokohama in 1871. In the ensuing decades all aspects of German medicine flowed into Japan; there has never been an instance in history where a country not under colonial domination so completely adopted an outside system.

The leading role of medicine in the development of Western influences in Japan was enunciated by two eminent Japanese statesmen in 1915. They were entertaining Wallace Buttrick, Simon Flexner, and William Henry Welch, the members of a commission sent by The Rockefeller Foundation to study the future of medicine in China. Count Ōkuma, the premier of Japan, explained to them that "the Occidental part of Japanese civilization had begun with the introduction of Western medicine" (Flexner and Flexner, p. 399).

A leading nobleman, Baron Shibusawa, also emphasized the dominance of medicine. He described three phases in the development of Western influences in Japan and stated that the first and earliest phase had been the introduction of Western medicine.

There are two principal reasons why medicine was the medium for the introduction of Western culture into Japan. Sir George Sansom has cited one:

> . . . it is characteristic of the early stages of Western studies in Japan during the Tokugawa Shogunate that it was the companion sciences of inflicting wounds and healing them that attracted the attention of ambitious young *samurai*. Those who did not study the manufacture and use of lethal weapons devoted themselves to medicine and surgery. These and astronomy were the features of Western culture that appealed to their minds and it was only incidentally that they acquired some knowledge of other aspects of European culture [1962, p. 253].

A second reason, and one that deserves special emphasis, is the singular veneration that the Japanese people hold for medicine. They are uniquely conscious of minor aberrations from a complete sense of well-being; they place full reliance on medicine to prevent or correct such deviations. The complaint "I feel weak" is frequently volunteered even by robust university students. At times the Japanese seem to be unduly eager to proclaim weakness while members of other societies are unduly eager to proclaim vigor. The weakness is corrected by large doses of vitamin B, preferably administered by a parenteral route—and preferably intravenously.

Buxom ladies in stunning kimonos sip vitamin B elixirs from glass vials purchased on the railway platform as they await the super-high-speed train to take them on a three-hour journey in overstuffed chairs with padded footrests. The "need for B" is described charmingly by the Japanese author Junichirō Tanizaki in his famous novel *The Makioka Sisters*.

Self-medication has been a custom in Japan for many centuries. Itinerant dispensers go from door to door leaving a spectrum of medicines with the housewife. The peddler returns in a month, is reimbursed for the medicines that have been consumed, and restocks the family pharmacy. With the ready availability of drugs through health insurance programs and loose controls over prescription counters, this practice is now largely confined to rural areas. Every Japanese household is said to possess at least one hypodermic syringe.

The widely publicized "flu mask" is worn not only to lessen exposure to respiratory infections but as well to "purify" air that is cold, moist, or heavy. Bulky bandages for minor infections or abrasions are a frequent part of the Japanese costume.

It was to study Western medicine and to acquire drugs that the Japanese came to Deshima, even though they were usually required to serve as menials in order to gain entry. Thus, after the Dutch had been at Deshima for half a century, we find a high Japanese official commenting: "With the exception of medicines, we can dispense with everything that is brought us from abroad" (Titsingh, 1822, p. 28).

As soon as the interpreters had acquired a knowledge of the rudiments of Western medicine and the drugs used by the Dutch, they turned to the practice of medicine because there was such a demand for the new system—and for the new drugs.

We have noted Thunberg's report that in 1775 patients lined the roadside on the *hofreis*, some of whom had struggled long distances to be attended. The Deshima doctors responded to the enthusiasm of the Japanese for medicine, and, although some of them were little better than barber-surgeons, they were willing to teach. In part this may have been because their vanity was touched by the respect shown them by the Japanese.

Until the last quarter of the eighteenth century the rise of Western medicine was at best slow. Thus, coming to Japan at the end of the seventeenth century, Engelbert Kaempfer's major contribution was his massive documentation of the Japanese culture for the West. Arriving at the dawn of the *Rangaku* era, Thunberg stimulated the development of Linnaean botany, but his major contribution, like Kaempfer's, was to the West—through his collections and his high status in European scientific circles, which drew attention to his numerous publications on Japan. There were only a handful of Japanese with whom these two men could communicate.

The establishment by Japanese of active programs to teach Western medicine, beginning with Maeno and Sugita in the last quarter of the eighteenth century, gave great impetus to the rise of Western medicine. It was Philipp Franz von Siebold who was the key European figure in the rise of Western medicine in Japan. He arrived at a time when the fundamentals of Western medicine had been grasped by the *Rangakusha;* he taught the Japanese how to practice Western medicine. Thirty years after Siebold, Pompe van Meerdervoort was the first to show how the basic and clinical medical sciences could be fitted together into a single body of knowledge.

Of the three Western medical explorers of Japan, we can rank Engelbert Kaempfer as the leading author and explorer, Carl Pieter Thunberg as the leading scientist, and Siebold as the leading teacher—and the most dramatic personage. Pompe van Meerdervoort made a heroic contribution in establishing a medical school at Nagasaki. From the Japanese side, they are joined by a remarkable handful of *Rangakusha*—Sugita Gempaku, Maeno Ryōtaku, Ōtsuki Gentaku, Takano Chōei, and Ogata Kōan. These great men from the East and West, building on the deep interest of the Japanese in foreign knowledge with a special concern for medicine and health, were responsible for the pioneering and dominant role of medicine in the development of Western influences in Japan.

I

Correspondence between William II of Holland and the Shogun of Japan, A.D. 1844*

"We, William the Second by the Grace of God, King of the Netherlands, Prince of Orange and Nassau, Grand Duke of Luxemburg etc., write this our Royal letter with a faithful heart to our Friend, the very noble, most serene, and allpowerful sovereign of the great Empire of Japan, who has his seat in the Imperial Palace of Yedo, the abode of peace.

"May this epistle be duly delivered into the hands of our imperial friend and find him in good health and peace.

"More than two centuries ago by Imperial order of your Majesty's serene ancestor, the celebrated Gongen Ijejas, permission was granted to the Dutch to come with their trading ships to Japan; and in virtue of this Imperial order, the Dutch our subjects, are still received and treated with all kindness in Japan, and moreover the leading men in that

* This translation of the correspondence between the two heads of government is by D. C. Greene and appeared in *Transactions of the Asiatic Society of Japan* 24, pt. 4 (1907): 99–123.

trade have been granted the honor of paying homage in person to Your Majesty.

"This unfaltering goodwill exhibited towards our subjects fills us with kindly feelings towards Japan and the desire to do all that is possible for the furtherance of peace within Your Imperial Domain and for the prosperity of Your subjects.

"There never has been any correspondence between the sovereigns of the Netherlands and Japan. There was no necessity, for, commercial affairs and general news were communicated by the government which under our control rules over Batavia and all the Islands belonging to our Dominion in Asia.

"But now we feel drawn to terminate this silence. There are important matters worthy of communication. They do not concern the trade of our subjects with Japan, but the political interests of the Empire. They relate to matters worthy to be treated of between King and King.

"The future of Japan causes us much anxiety. May we succeed in averting imminent disaster by our good counsel.

"From the communications that our vessels bring from year to year to Nagasaki, Your Majesty will have learnt that the King of England has lately been waging a violent war against the Chinese Empire.

"The mighty Emperor of China after a long but fruitless resistance, was finally compelled to succumb to the superior power of European military tactics, and in the consequent treaty of peace, agreed to conditions by which the ancient Chinese policy has undergone great alteration, and whereby five Chinese ports have been opened to European trade.

"When, thirty years ago, the war which had been waged in Europe, was terminated, all nations began to work for peace.

"The Kings remembering the lesson of the wise opened to their subjects every channel for trade.

"Populations were on the increase. The discoveries in machinery and physics rendered manual labor less necessary.

"Commerce and industry rapidly increased everywhere, but, nevertheless, there was in many countries, a lack of the necessities of life.

"This was especially the case in mighty England, notwithstanding the wealth, the resources and the enterprising spirit of the inhabitants. Restlessly seeking new channels for their trade, in their efforts to do so, they sometimes came in conflict with foreign nations. The English Government by force of circumstances was then compelled to assist and protect its subjects by force.

"In this way quarrels occurred between the English merchants and the Chinese officials at Canton. From that quarrel war arose. That war was fatal to China, for many thousand Chinese were killed, many cities were taken and devastated, many millions in treasure were yielded as indemnity to the conquerors.

"Such disasters now threaten the Japanese Empire. A mere mischance might precipitate a conflict. The number of all sorts of vessels sailing the Japanese seas will be greater than ever before, and how easily might a quarrel occur between the crews of those vessels and the inhabitants of Your Majesty's Dominion.

"The thought that such quarrels may end in war fills us with solicitude. The wisdom that characterises your Majesty's Government will, we hope, know how to avert these dangers.

"This wisdom was already evident in the mandate, which was read by the Government of Nagasaki to the Netherlands Supreme Official on the thirteenth of the eighth month of the year 1842, ordering the kindly treatment of all foreign vessels. But is that mandate sufficient?

"Only such vessels are mentioned, as are driven on to the Japanese coast by hurricane or lack of provisions. What will be done with vessels that come for other and friendly reasons to visit the Japanese coast?

"Are these to be repulsed by force or unfriendly treatment? Will quarrels arise? Quarrels lead to war, and war leads to destruction. Those are the disasters which we wish to avert from Japan. It is our desire as a token of gratefulness for the hospitality enjoyed by our subjects for more than two hundred years. The philosopher says: 'In security, we must guard against danger; in peace, against confusion.'

"We have watched the course of events with serious attention. The intercourse between the different nations of the earth is increasing with great rapidity. An irresistible power is drawing them together. Through the invention of steamships distances have become shorter. A nation preferring to remain in isolation at this time of increasing relationships could not avoid hostility with many others.

"We know that the laws of Your Majesty's serene Ancestors were issued with a view rigorously to restrict intercourse with foreign nations. But (says Lao Tseu) 'when wisdom is seated on the throne, she will excel in maintaining peace.' When in the strict observance of old laws, peace might be disturbed, wisdom will succeed in smoothing difficulties.

"This, Allpowerful Emperor, is our friendly advice, ameliorate the laws against the foreigners, lest happy Japan be destroyed by war. We give Your Majesty this advice with honest intentions, free from political self-interest.

"We hope that wisdom will make the Japanese Government realise that peace can only be maintained through friendly relations, and that these are only created by commercial relations.

"Should Your Majesty be desirous of receiving further information in this matter so important for Japan, then we shall be pleased, after receiving a letter from Your Majesty's own hand, to send an Envoy to Japan, one who possesses our entire confidence, and who might be able to explain to Your Majesty all particulars which we have roughly outlined in this letter.

"While we are anxious about the happiness and peace of far off Japan, we ourselves are weighed down with grief, for it has pleased providence to summon recently our beloved father, King William the First, who had retired from the care of political affairs four years ago, after bearing their burden for twenty-eight years. We are convinced of Your Majesty's sympathy in our lawful sorrow.

"We send this letter by one of our men-of-war, hoping that the same will bring an answer from Your Majesty. In that vessel is our portrait which we wish to present to Your Majesty as a token of our sincere friendship. That vessel will also bring certain presents for Your Majesty as noted on the accompanying list. They are of little value and consist of reproductions of Industry, Art and Science, flourishing under our patronage in the Netherlands.

"For the courtesy continually shown to our subjects, we offer You our thanks. We further commend them to the protection of the Japanese Government.

"We wish Your Majesty, that the Almighty, who blessed Your serene Father with so long a reign, will permit Your Majesty to enjoy the same prosperity. May blessing, rest, and peace be granted to the great Empire of Japan for all time.

"Given at our Royal Palace at The Hague the 15th day of February 1844, in the fourth year of our reign."

[Signed] William

The Minister of Colonies
[Signed] J. C. Baud

The Emperor (?) of Japan to the King of Holland

"I, Emperor and King of Japan, wish to the King of Holland (Prince of Orange) who hath sent from so far countries to visit me, greeting.

"I rejoice greatly in your writing and sending unto me, and wish that our countries were nearer the one to the other, whereby we might continue and increase the friendship begun betwixt us, through your presence, whom I imagine in earnest to see; in respect I am unknown unto Your Majesty and that your love towards me is manifested through your liberality in honoring me with four presents, whereof, though I had no need, yet coming in Your name, I received them in great worth and hold them in good esteem.

"And further, whereas the Hollanders, Your Majesty's subjects, desire to trade with their shipping in my country (which is of little value and small), and to traffic with my subjects, and desire to have their abiding near unto my court, whereby in person I might help and assist them, which can not be as now, through the inconvenience of the country; yet, notwithstanding, I will not neglect, as already I have been, to be careful of them and to give in charge to all my governors and subjects that, in what places and havens, in what port soever, they shall show them all favour and friendships to their persons, ships and merchandise; wherein Your Majesty or your subjects need not to doubt or fear aught to the contrary. For they may come as freely as if they come into Your Majesty's own havens and countries, and so may remain in my country to trade. And the friendship begun between me and my subjects with you shall never be impaired on my behalf, but augmented and increased.

"I am partly ashamed that Your Majesty (whose name and renown through your valorous deeds is spread through the whole world) should cause your subjects to come from so far countries into a country so unfitting as this is, to visit me and to offer unto me such friendships as I have not deserved. But considering that your affection hath been the cause thereof, I could not but friendly entertain your subjects, and yield to their requests, whereof this shall serve for a testimony, that they in all places, countries, and islands, under mine obedience, may trade and traffic, and build houses serviceable and needful for their trade and merchandises, where they may trade without any hindrance at their pleasure, as well in time to come as for the present, so that no man shall do them any wrong. And I will defend and maintain them as my own subjects.

"I promise, likewise, that the persons whom I understand shall be left here, shall now and at all times be held as recommended unto me, and in all things to favour them whereby Your Majesty shall find us as your friends and neighbours.

"For other matters passed between me and Your Majesty's servants, which would be too long here to repeat, I refer myself to them."

Chronology of the Rise of Western Medicine in Japan

A.D.

414   Kon Mu of Silla, a kingdom in southeast Korea, invited to serve as physician to emperor of Japan.

King of Paekche, another Korean kingdom, sent a group of scholars, including physicians, to Japan.

458 (?) Body of Princess Takuhata autopsied by order of imperial writ.

552   Buddhism officially introduced into Japan from Korea.
(or 538) Teachers of Chinese medicine bearing Chinese medical texts came to Japan from Paekche.

602   Priest-physician, Kwan Roku, came to Japan and taught Chinese medicine.

608   First Japanese medical students sent to China for study.

702   Taihō Law Code called for establishment of medical schools and colleges in capital city and each prefecture but was never promulgated.

712 (?)   *Kojiki* compiled.

720 (?)   *Nihon Shoki* compiled.

730   Hospital established in Nara, the capital city.

735   First smallpox epidemic officially recorded.

794   Kyoto founded.

808   *Daido-Mijuho*, a text on Japanese indigenous medicine, compiled.

982   *Ishinho* compiled.

1303   Kajiwara Shozun published *Man-anpo*, an anatomical text.

1494   Treaty of Tordesillas included Japan in half of world allocated to Portuguese with exclusive rights to trade and spread Christianity.

1498   Tashiro Sanki introduced *Ri-shū* system of medicine from China. Vasco da Gama opened sea road to India.

1542–43 Portuguese sailors blown ashore at Tanegashima.

1549   St. Francis Xavier arrived in Japan.

1550   Manase Dōsan stimulated spread of *Ri-shū* school across southern Japan.

1555   Luis d'Almeida, Lisbon surgeon, first Western doctor to practice in Japan.

1565   First edict to expel Jesuits issued but not enforced.

1568   Oda Nobunaga seized Kyoto and permitted Jesuits to practice Western medicine and surgery at Nambanji Temple.

1574   Manase Dōsan published *Keiteki-shū*, a compilation of old Japanese medical texts and theories.

1582   Practice of medicine by Jesuits restricted by Alexander Valignano, visitor-general.

1587   New decree issued for expulsion of Christian missionaries.

1593   Spanish friars, principally Franciscans from Manila, established missions and hospitals in Japan.

1595   First Dutch fleets entered Asian waters.

1597   Twenty-six Christian martyrs—nine European Franciscans and seventeen converts—crucified at Nagasaki.

1609   Dutch established trading post on Hirado Island.

1613   English established factory on Hirado.
        Pen-ts'ao Kang-mu, Chinese book on botany and natural history, brought to Japan.

1614   Edict expelling all priests from Japan strictly enforced.

1622–23 Period of greatest persecution of Christians.

1623   English abandoned Hirado factory.
        Apostate Jesuit physician, Cristavão Ferreira, who later took the name Sawano, wrote *Nambanryū geka-sho*, a book on Portuguese surgery.

1624   All Spaniards expelled from Japan.

1633–36 Edicts for *sakoku* ("closed country") issued; included ban on books.

1636   Deshima built in Nagasaki Bay; remaining Portuguese traders moved there.

1638   Last Portuguese traders expelled.

1641   Dutch moved from Hirado Island to Deshima.
        First factory doctor, Juriaen Henseelingh, arrived at Deshima.
        Japan closed to all Western contacts except the Dutch at Deshima.

1647   Willem Ten Rhijne born in Deventer, The Netherlands.

1649   Caspar Schamberger practiced and taught Western surgery on Deshima and in Edo.

1651   Engelbert Kaempfer born in Lemgo, Germany.

1665   Certificate of proficiency in Dutch medicine and surgery issued to Japanese student at Deshima.

1674   Willem Ten Rhijne arrived at Deshima.

1683   Ten Rhijne published first description of techniques and uses of acupuncture and moxibustion for the West.

1690   Engelbert Kaempfer came to Deshima.
Motoki Ryōi began translation of German anatomy textbook by Johannes Rommelin (not published until 1772).

1700   Willem Ten Rhijne died.

1712   Kaempfer's *Amoenitatum Exoticarum* published.

1716   Nagasaki trade with Dutch limited to two ships each year.
Kaempfer died at Lemgo.

1720   Tokugawa Yoshimune lifted ban on books to permit circulation of books that did not contain Christian doctrine.

1723   Maeno Ryōtaku born.

1727   Kaempfer's *The History of Japan* published under auspices of Sir Hans Sloane.

1733   Sugita Gempaku born.

1740   Aoki Konyō and Noro Genjō commissioned to learn the Dutch alphabet by Shogun Tokugawa Yoshimune.

1743   Carl Pieter Thunberg born.

1745   First Dutch dictionary compiled by Aoki Konyō.

1754   Yamawaki Tōyō, a physician of the Kohō school of *Kampō*, recorded in *Zōshi* the first objective findings from a human dissection.

1757   Ōtsuki Gentaku, father of Dutch scholarship, born.

1759   Founding of British Museum in London and deposition of Kaempfer collections there.
Kuriyama Kōan, pupil of Yamawaki Tōyō, performed first dissection of female cadaver.

1771   Sugita Gempaku and Maeno Ryōtaku observed human dissection and found that the anatomy agreed with that described in a Western compendium, *Anatomische Tabellen*.

1772   *Oranda zenku Naigai bungō Zu*, translation of German anatomical text, published.

1773   Maeno and Sugita prepare *Kaitai Yakuzu*, a preliminary text on Western anatomy; published in Sugita's name only.

1774   *Kaitai Shinsho*, a translation of Kulmus' *Anatomische Tabellen*, published by Sugita and colleagues.

1775   Thunberg came to Deshima and introduced new Linnaean botany to Japan.

1783   *Rangaku Kaitei*, a Dutch grammar, translated into Japanese by Ōtsuki Gentaku.

1784   Thunberg's *Flora Japonica* published.

1786   Ōtsuki opened Shirandō, first private school for the study of Western medicine and Dutch.

1788   Ōtsuki published *Rangaku Kaitei* [Ladder to the Dutch studies].

1790   Sugita Gempaku and Ōtsuki Gentaku published *Yōi Shinsho*, a translation from the Dutch edition of Heister's *Chirurgie*.

1793   Udagawa Genzui's translation of Johannes de Gorter's *Medicinae-compendium* the first Japanese text on internal medicine.
Katsuragawa Hoshū appointed surgeon to *bakufu*.

1796   Inamura Sanpaku published the dictionary *Halma Wage*.
Philipp Franz Balthasar von Siebold born in Würzburg, Germany.

1803   Maeno Ryōtaku died.

1805   *Ihan Teikō*, textbook of Western anatomy and physiology, published by Udagawa Genshin.

1809–17 Holland seized by Napoleon; Batavia taken by the British.

1810   Ogata Kōan born.

1813   *Oranda Kyokuhō*, text on Western pharmacy and pharmacology, published by Udagawa Genshin.

1817   Sugita Gempaku died.

1822–23 Thunberg's *Fauna Japonica* published.

1823   Siebold came to Deshima.

213

1824   Siebold began to teach Western medicine and natural science on the mainland at Nagasaki.

1826   Siebold made *hofreis* to Edo and acquired the Great Map of Japan.

1827   Ōtsuki Gentaku died.

1828   Thunberg died.
Ship bearing Siebold's purloined collection wrecked in a typhoon.
Udagawa Genshin published *Oranda Yakkyō*, a text on European materia medica.

1829   Siebold banished for possessing maps of Japan.
J. L. C. Pompe van Meerdervoort born.

1832–41 Siebold's books *Flora Japonica*, *Fauna Japonica*, and *Nippon* published.

1836   Takano Chōei published *Igen suyō*, first modern physiology text in Japan.

1837   Ogata Kōan opened Tekiteki-sai Juku at Osaka.
National Ethnographic Museum housing Siebold collection established in Leiden.

1838   Satō Taizen began to teach Western medicine at Edo.

1839   Takano Chōei imprisoned.

1840   All Western studies, except medicine, banned.

1844   William II of The Netherlands dispatched a letter to Tokugawa Ieyoshi.

1845   Siebold opened botanical garden near Leiden.

1847   Ogata Kōan published first Western pathology text, *Byōgaku (Byori) Tsūron*.

1849   Otto Mohnike, a factory doctor, introduced vaccination against smallpox.
Ban on Western studies extended to medicine.

1850   Takano Chōei committed *seppuku*.

1852   Siebold sought appointment to Perry expedition; visited Russia.

1853   Commodore Matthew C. Perry arrived at Uraga.

1856   Shogun requested Dutch to send a frigate, and a Dutch doctor to teach at Nagasaki.

1857   Pompe van Meerdervoort arrived at Nagasaki and established first Western medical school in Japan.

1858   Vaccination Institute established at Edo, forerunner of Tokyo Imperial University Medical School.
        Future Keio University founded by Fukuzawa Yukichi.
        Six Western-trained doctors appointed as physicians to shogun.

1859   Dr. J. C. Hepburn, American medical missionary and scholar, arrived in Japan.
        Siebold returned to Japan.
        Pompe van Meerdervoort given first body for dissection.

1861   New medical school building and teaching hospital completed at Nagasaki.
        Name of Vaccination Institute at Edo changed to Institute of Western Medicine; instruction in Western medicine began.

1862   Pompe van Meerdervoort returned to Holland.
        Ogata Kōan assumed position as director of Institute for Western Medicine in Edo.

1863   Siebold left Japan at request of Dutch ambassador.
        Ogata Kōan died.

1866   Philipp Franz Balthasar von Siebold died.

1867   Meiji enthroned as emperor; shogunate overthrown.
        First body willed for dissection.

1867–68   *Vijf Jaren in Japan* published by Pompe van Meerdervoort.

1870   Decision made to adopt German system of medicine; German medical teachers asked to come to Tokyo.
        Twelve students sent to Germany for medical training.

1871   Drs. Leopold Mueller, Prussian army surgeon, and Theodore Hoffmann, Prussian navy surgeon, arrived in Tokyo to organize new program of medical education at Tokyo University.

1908   J. L. C. Pompe van Meerdervoort died.

Glossary

ANMA-SEI——Literally, massage student. A highly stylized technique of massage has been popular in Japan for more than a millennium. Historically, as today, the masseurs were usually blind.

BAKUFU——Literally, curtain office or tent government. Originally the camp of the shogun in the field of battle, but later the shogunate. It included all of the governmental, administrative, and military offices staffed by retainers of the Tokugawa.

BONZES——A popular term applied to all Buddhist priests. Today the usual term is *bōsan* or *bōzu*.

BUGYŌ——Literally, perform the given order. A term applied to magistrates and chief administrators or more loosely to ministers of state, secretaries, judges, and local and municipal administrators.

CHŌME——A sequential distance. Section of a city such as 1-chōme.

CHUNG-I——Literally, medicine of China. Referred to today as Chinese traditional medicine, it is based on the belief that health is dependent upon the maintenance of *yin* and *yang*, the opposing forces of the universe. For more than a millennium it was the base of Japanese medicine, which was termed *Kampō*.

DAIGAKU——Literally, great learning. The term for a university.

DAIMYŌ——Literally, great name. In feudal Japan, a lord who ruled a feudatory and held the unswerving allegiance of his knights, who would pay with their lives to avenge his dishonor.

217

DESHIMA (OR DEJIMA)——Literally, going-out island. An artificial island in Nagasaki Bay on which for more than two centuries the Japanese permitted the Dutch to maintain a small trading post. During this period, Deshima was the seat of contact between Japan and the West.

EDO——Literally, bay door. Until the Meiji Restoration in 1868, the seat of the military ruler. When Meiji moved the throne to Edo, the name was changed to Tokyo.

EDO PERIOD——Period of the Tokugawa shogunate.

ETA——Literally, full of dirt. Orginally, *etori*, meaning a person who gathered bait for the dogs and hawks of nobles. The name of a pariah caste, the members of which slaughtered cattle and worked with hides. Shunned by their fellowmen, they were called upon to perform the periodic dismemberments of beheaded criminals.

FUGU——Literally, river pig. Globe-fish, a highly popular delicacy in Japan today. The liver and ovaries contain a highly toxic material, a tetrodotoxin which may be lethal, and the fish must be cleaned meticulously before human consumption.

FUMIYE——Literally, step on picture. Trampling on a metal plate bearing an image of the Virgin Mary and the cross. This ritual was required of every citizen on the New Year to show his contempt for Christianity.

FŪSETSUSHO——Literally, wind snow book (annual report). The Dutch were required to report to the shogun each year on the state of the countries with which they traded and the activities of the Portuguese.

GEHEIMRAT——Literally, secret councilor to the throne. Used today to describe an imperious, autocratic professor.

GEISHA——Literally, artistic performing person. A professional entertainer who has received formal training as a *maiko* in traditional dancing, singing, and playing classical musical instruments; her primary role is to provide charming companionship. She is not a prostitute in the usual connotation, and any sexual relationship is only by mutual consent, with arrangements approved by a female to whom the geisha owes complete loyalty. The world of the geisha is the most feudal aspect of Japanese society today.

GENKAN——Literally, mysterious gate. Originally the entrance or gate to a Zen temple. Now applied to the entrance hall in a Japanese home.

GENROKU ERA (1688–1704)——The height of opulence in the Edo period, characterized by prosperity and creativity in intellectual pursuits and the creative arts.

HAIKU——Traditional Japanese poems of seventeen syllables with a key word indicating the season. They are of Buddhist origin and usually reflect the Buddhist view of the illusory and transitory endless cycle of life. However, some are amusing and witty. The poems are impressionistic and merely suggest images; there are no concrete descriptions.

218

HAKAMA——Divided skirt. A part of the traditional costume of Japanese males on occasions of ceremony, such as marriages, funerals, and ancestral rites. Often made of silk, it is worn with a stiff coat called a *haori*. Historically the *hakama* could only be worn by *daimyō* or samurai with a *kamishimo* on top.

HITOYOGIRI——Literally, one-joint cutting. A musical instrument like a *shakuhachi*, but made from a single section of bamboo.

HOFREIS——High trip. Annual journey by the *opperhoofd*, the doctor, and other foreigners to Edo to report to the shogun on affairs in the West.

HONZŌ-GAKU——Literally, plant study. The study of plants for medicinal purposes. Also botany.

ISE SHRINE——Ise is actually the name of a province applied to the two *Jingū* shrines which are the seat of Shinto near the town of Yamada. They are remarkably simple in design and by immemorial custom must be razed and rebuilt every twenty years with no change in style.

JAMMABOS (OR YAMABUSHI)——Literally, mountain priest. A Buddhist sect, aggressively combative and independent, and openly defiant of the government. Its headquarters were on Mt. Hiei, north of Kyoto; it is the guardian mountain for the former imperial city.

JŌRURI——A ballad-drama acted out through the use of puppets.

KABUKI——Literally, to sing and dance. A highly stylized variety of theater with elaborate costumes and scenery. All roles are taken by men. Historically a half-religious and half-erotic entertainment in one style of which, *Onna Kabuki*, all parts were played by females; in another style, *Wakashū Kabuki*, all parts were played by boys.

KAITŌ——Literally, answer.

KAKEMONO——Literally, hanging thing. An art scroll which is hung in a recessed area in a Japanese home and is changed periodically. It usually depicts the season, such as cherry blossoms in the spring, red maple leaves in the autumn, and cranes at the New Year.

KAMBUN——Literally, Han writing. Written in Chinese characters (*kanji*), this was the preferred language of Japanese scholars.

KAMPŌ——Literally, Han technique. The Japanese name for the traditional medicine brought from China. *Kam* or *Kan* is the Japanese name for the Han dynasty of China, the period in which Chinese medical arts first came to Japan.

KANJI——Han characters.

KANSAI——Literally, western area of the barrier. The plain which includes Kyoto, Osaka, and Kobe.

KANTŌ——Literally, eastern area of the barrier. The plain which includes the Tokyo area.

KARŌ——Councilor of the clan. Men of varied talents, of no established number, who directed the feudatories under the *daimyō*.

219

KIMONO——Literally, something to wear. The traditional garment of Japan.

KŌJA (OR GYŌJA)——Buddhist priests from a mountain near Kyoto who, unlike priests of other orders, were allowed to travel freely.

KOKUGAKU——Literally, nation's studies (provincial schools). Proposed under the Taihō Code but never accomplished.

KŌMŌ——Literally, red hairs. The name given to the Hollanders to illustrate their sinister nature rather than the actual color of their hair. The Japanese almost invariably portrayed the Hollanders with red hair.

MEIJI RESTORATION——In 1868 Mutsuhito who had been enthroned as the Emperor Meiji in the preceding year was restored to the role of the true ruler, the office of Shogun was abolished, and the seat of government was moved from Kyoto to Tokyo. During this era, Japan set itself upon a course to adopt Western patterns of government and education.

MIKADO——Literally, great place or august gate. The term is used to denote the heaven-descended emperor who represents the oldest reigning family in the world, although succession has not followed strict rules of legitimacy.

NIHONBASHI——Literally, Nippon Bridge. The most famous bridge in Japan. It marked the start of the Tōkaido road, which ended at Sanjo Bridge in Kyoto. All distances in Japan were measured from Nihonbashi.

NOH (OR NŌ) THEATER——Classic play in which actors wear expressionless but imaginatively carved masks. All emotions are portrayed by the actions of actors, speeches are chanted, and the audience usually follows the text in a book. Musicians and a chorus are used to comment on the characters and describe scenes. The emphasis of the play is on beauty more than on any theme or "message." Classic language and costumes, sparse, imaginative settings, a chorus, the stately bearing of actors who are often masked—these suggest old Greek drama. *Noh* was basically aristocratic entertainment while *Kabuki* was for the common people.

NORIMON——Literally, riding things. Palanquin.

Ō-NA-MUCHI-NO-MIKOTO——One of the two semideities to which the origins of medicine are attributed. God of Izumo Shrine.

ORANDA——Holland.

ORANDA-Ō-ME——Literally, Dutch-big-eyes. One term which Japanese children applied to the Hollanders. The large round eyes of the foreigners impressed them as a sign of their demonic character.

OTTOMAN PORTE——Literally, Ottoman High Gate. The chief office of the Ottoman Empire.

RANGAKU——Literally, Dutch study. The term applied to the period from 1774 to the opening of Japan to the West.

RANGAKUSHA——Literally, Dutch study person. Term applied to those who were engaged in the study of Dutch, Dutch medicine and science, and mathematics.

RI——Japanese measure of distance equal to three kilometers.

RINKŌ——Reading and explaining class.

RŌJU——Literally, among the old. The council of elders which was the senior and the most powerful body in the *bakufu*.

RŌNIN——Literally, floating person. Name applied to the numerous masterless samurai. In modern parlance, a student who has failed the university entrance examinations and is awaiting another try.

RYOKAN——Literally, traveler's house. A hotel or inn.

SAKE——Japanese rice wine which is used when making a toast at significant events as well as for pleasure.

SAKOKU——Literally, chained country. The centuries during which Japan was closed to the West.

SAMURAI——Literally, loyal servant. The knights of feudal Japan whose unique right was permission to carry a sword, but who were completely dependent upon their lord, the *daimyō*.

SENRYŪ POEMS——Literally, river willow. Satirical poems written in colloquial or spoken language. They contain the same number of syllables as haiku, but are more frivolous and not as seriously and carefully written. Occasionally *Senryū* poems carried the message of a social or political protest.

SENSEI——Literally, born before. Any teacher, not necessarily an academic person.

SEPPUKU——Literally, cut in belly. The traditional method of suicide with a short dagger. *Seppuku* was a moral obligation for a samurai to retain personal honor if he failed to follow social codes, lacked personal courage, or had not completely fulfilled his responsibilities. Also referred to as hara-kiri, for which the same characters are used but in reverse order.

SHINTO——Literally, way of the gods. A collection of traditions, rituals, pilgrimages, and shrines emphasizing nature and ancestor worship. There is no systematic philosophy or well-defined moral code characteristic of the usual religion, but Shinto has always included the worship of the emperor as a direct descendant of the sun goddess Amaterasu, who, according to legend, founded Japan. Re-emphasized and pronounced a state religion by the militarist regimes in the years preceding World War II, it became a rallying point for zealous nationalists. Shinto was abolished as an organ of the state in 1946, and today its shrines are used primarily for a brief prayer and its priests for ceremonies comparable to baptisms and weddings. Any official event may be opened with a Shinto ritual.

SHŌGATSU——Literally, the correct month. The first month of the year and Japan's most important holiday. Officially the first three days in

January. All debts must be paid, and gifts termed *seibo* are exchanged before *Shōgatsu*.

SHOGUN——The abbreviation for *Seiitaishōgun*. Literally, barbarian-killing general. Historically the title could only be given by the emperor to the military and administrative leader. The title was first granted in 1192 and was abolished in 1867 with the fall of the Tokugawa regime. During this period the emperor continued his court in Kyoto but was powerless.

SHOSHIDAI——A powerful magistrate who protected the emperor's palace in Kyoto, supervised clans west of Kyoto, and governed civil administration in the Kinki area during the Edo period.

SUICHIKU-IN——Literally, green bamboo garden. Honorific title given to Manase Dōsan.

SUKUNA-HIKONA-NO-MIKOTO——One of the two semideities to which the origins of medicine are attributed (see *Ō-na-muchi-no-mikoto*).

T'ANG DYNASTY——This regime brought China to the position of the richest, most-powerful, most-opulent, and best-governed country in the world. It was during this period that Japan turned to China and borrowed heavily from her rich storehouse of culture.

TATAMI——Literally, folding. The rush mats made from *Juncus effusus* which cover the floor of a Japanese-style room.

TŌKAIDO——Literally, eastern sea road. Japan's most famous road, which stretches from Edo to Kyoto. There were fifty-three ordained stops memorialized in the prints of Hiroshige.

TOKONOMA——Literally, space of floor. A recessed area or alcove in a Japanese home. In addition to the *kakemono*, it may contain family treasures, ornamental vases, and floral bouquets. An honored guest is always seated before the *tokonoma*.

TOKYO——Literally, eastern capital. The name applied to the capital city of Edo after the Meiji Restoration in 1868.

TYCOON——Literally, great emperor or sovereign. The name applied by Western visitors to the rulers of Japan and of China.

Bibliography

Ackerknecht, E. H. 1955. *A short history of medicine.* New York: The Ronald Press Co.

————. 1957. Medical education in 19th century France. *Journal Med. Ed.* 32: 148–52.

————. 1967. *Medicine at the Paris hospital, 1794–1848.* Baltimore: The Johns Hopkins Press.

Adams, F. O. 1874. *The history of Japan.* London: H. S. King and Co.

Alcock, Sir R. A. 1863. *Capital of the tycoon.* 2 vols. New York: Harper and Bros.

Aston, W. G. 1896. Nihonogi, chronicles of Japan, from the earliest time to A.D. 697. *Transactions of Proceedings of Japan Society*, Supplement no. 1. 2 vols. London: Kegan Paul, Trench, Trubner and Co.

Backer, Augustin de. 1890–1932. *Bibliothèque de la Compagnie de Jésus.* New ed., 1: 195–96. Brussels: Carlos Sommervogel.

Banks, Sir Joseph. 1791. *Icones selectae Plantarum quas in Japonien collegit et delineavit E. Kaempfer ex archetypis in Museo Britannico Asservatis.* 59 plates. London.

Bijleveld, M. 1932. *Von Siebold: Bijdragen tot zine levensbeschrijving.* Leiden: Siebold Collection, Rijksmuseum.

Billroth, Theodor. 1924. *The medical sciences in the German universities: A study in the history of civilization.* New York: Macmillan Co.

223

Blok, Petrus Johannes. 1907. Frederick Henry, John De Witt, William III. *History of the people of The Netherlands*, pt. 4. Translated by Oscar A. Bierstadt. New York: G. P. Putnam's Sons; London: Knickerbocker Press.

Bourdon, Léon. 1949. Luis de Almeida, chirurgien et marchand avant son entrée dans la Compagnie de Jésus au Japon, 1525(?)–1556. Thesis in *Mélanges d'études portugaises offerts à M. Georges Le Gentil*, pp. 69–85. Lisbon.

Bowers, J. Z. 1965. *Medical Education in Japan*. New York: Harper & Row.

———. 1966. Engelbert Kaempfer: Physician, explorer, scholar, and author. *Journal Hist. Med.* 21: 237–59.

Boxer, C. R. 1950. *Jan Compagnie in Japan, 1600–1850*. 2d rev. ed. The Hague: Martinus Nijhoff.

———. 1959. *The great ship from Amacon: Annals of Macao and the old Japan trade, 1555–1640*. Reprint, 1963. Lisbon: Centro de Estudos Historicos Ultramarinos.

———. 1965. *The Dutch sea-borne empire: 1600–1800*. New York: Alfred A. Knopf.

———. 1967. *The Christian century in Japan, 1549–1650*. Berkeley and Los Angeles: University of California Press.

Boyer, Samuel Pellman. 1963. *Naval surgeon, revolt in Japan, 1868–1869: The diary of Samuel Pellman Boyer*. Edited by Elinor and James A. Barnes. Introduction by Allan Nevins. Bloomington: Indiana University Press.

Bretschneider, Emil. 1898. *History of European botanical discoveries in China, London and St. Petersburg*. London: Sampson Low, Marston & Co.

Breynius, J. 1678. Excerpta ex observationibus Japonicis de fructice thee, cum fasciculo rarium plantarum ab ipso in Promontorio Bonae Spei et Sardhana sinu anno 1673 collectarum atque demum ex India anno 1677 in Europan ab Jacobus Breynius transmissarum, by Willem Ten Rhijne. *Exoticarum Plantarum Centuria prima*. Danzig.

Broes van Dort, T. 1898. *Historische studie over Lepra, Zoornanelijk in Verband: Met Het Zoor Komen Dezerziekt in Nederlandische Oost-Indie*. Rotterdam: W. J. van Hengel; Batavia: G. Kolff and Co.

Busk, W., ed. 1841. *Manners and customs of the Japanese in the nineteenth century: From recent Dutch visitors of Japan and the German of Dr. Ph. Fr. von Siebold*. London: John Murray.

Caron, F. 1663. *A true description of the mighty kingdoms of Japan and Siam*. Translated by Captain R. Manley. London.

Chabrie, R. 1933. Michel Boym, Jesuits, Polonais, etc. *Notices Biographiques et Bibliographiques*. Paris.

Chamberlain, Basil H. 1882. The Kojiki or record of ancient matters. *Transactions of the Asiatic Society of Japan*, vol. 10, supplement.

————. 1891. *Things Japanese*. Revised and enlarged edition. London: Kegan Paul, Trench, Trubner and Co.

Chinese therapeutical methods of acupuncture and moxibustion. 1962. Peking: Foreign Language Press.

Churchill, A., and Churchill, J. 1774. An account of the Cape of Good Hope and the Hottentots, the natives of that country with some animadversions upon the same by Henry Secreta a Zevoszit, by Willem Ten Rhijne, printed at Schaffhausen, Switzerland. *A collection of voyages and travels, some now first printed from original manuscripts, others now first published in English . . . with a general preface giving an account on the progress of navigation, from its first beginning.* 3d ed. London.

Cleyer, Andreas. 1682. *Specimen Medicinae Sinicae Nive Opuscula Medica ad Mentem Sinensium Continens: I–De Pulsibus Libros quatuor e sinico translatos, II–Tractatus de Pulsibus ad eruditio Europaeo collectos, III–Fragmentum Operis Medici ibidem ab eruditio Europaeo conscripti, IV–Excerpta Literis eruditi Europaei in China, V–Schematica ad meliorem prosecedentium Intelligentiam, VI–De Indiciis Morborum ex Linguae coloribus & affectionibus.* Frankfurt: Johannes Petrus.

————. 1695. *Flora Japonica Sive Flores Herbarum Arborum praecipui totius fere vasti Insularum Imperii Asiatici, Japan dicti, ab ipsis barbaris incolis Japanensibus ad viva florum exemplaria coloribus suis nativis penicillo depicti, apositis suis Japanensium characteribus & nominibus, a Clariss,* vol. 2. Two volumes of the manuscript are presently located at the Stiftung Preussischen Kulturbesitz Bibliothek, Marburg.

Cocks, Richard. 1883. *The diary of Richard Cocks, cape-merchant in the English factory in Japan, 1612–1622.* Edited by E. M. Thompson. 2 vols. London.

Cole, Allan B. 1947. *Yankee surveyors in the shogun's seas: Records of the United States surveying expedition to the North Pacific Ocean, 1853–1856.* Princeton: Princeton University Press.

Cooper, Michael, S.J., ed. 1965. *They came to Japan: An anthology of European reports on Japan, 1543–1640.* London: Thames and Hudson.

Costa Santos, Sebastião. 1925. O início da Escola de Cirurgia do Hospital Real de Todos os Santos, 1504–1565. Faculdade de Medicina de Lisboa, Primeiro Centenário Da Fundaçáo da Régia Escola de Cirurgia de Lisboa, 1825–1925. Lisbon.

Crawley, C. W., ed. 1965. *War and peace in an age of upheaval, 1793–1830.* The New Cambridge Modern History, vol. 9. Cambridge.

Croizier, Ralph C. 1968. *Traditional medicine in modern China: Science, nationalism and the tensions of cultural change.* Cambridge: Harvard University Press.

Cross, John. 1815. *Sketches of the medical school of Paris.* London.

Dandy, J. E., ed. 1958. *The Sloane Herbarium: An annotated list of the Horti Sicci composing it; with biographical accounts of the principal contributors,* pp. 144–45. London: Balding & Mansell.

Daudet, Alphonse. 1913. *Contes du Lundi.* New edition, revised and enlarged. Edited by Eugene Fasquelle. Paris: Bibliothèque-Charpentier.

de Beer, G. R. 1953. *Sir Hans Sloane and the British Museum.* Oxford.

de Morant, G. Soulie. 1934. *Précis de la Vraie Acuponcture Chinoise: Doctrine, Diagnostique, Thérapeutique.* Paris: Mercure de France.

Doeff, Hendrik. 1833. *Herringen uit Japan van Hendrik Doeff, Ridder der Orde van den Nederlandschen Leeuw, oud Opperhoofd Der Nederlanders in Japan op het Eiland Decima.* Haarlem: De Erven Francois Bohn.

Dore, R. P. 1965. *Education in Tokugawa Japan.* Berkeley and Los Angeles: University of California Press.

Dorssen, J. M. H. van. 1911. Willem Ten Rhijne (geb. te Deventer 1647, overl. te Batavia 1 Juni 1700). *Geneesk. Tijdschr. v. Nederl. Indie* 51, sec. 2.

Engelbert Kaempfer, sa vie, ses écrits, ses voyages. *Variétes Orientales,* pp. 98–122. 1865; 3d ed., 1872.

Esso, I. van. 1941. Die Medizinischen Beziehungen Zwischen Japan Und Holland (Im 17, 18 und 19 Jahrhundert). *Janus* 45: 114–36.

Fairbank, John K.; Reischauer, Edwin O.; and Craig, Albert M. 1965. *East Asia, the modern transformation.* Boston: Houghton Mifflin Co.

Falkmann, ———. 1882. *Allgemeine Deutsche Biographie,* vol. 15. Munich and Leipzig: Dunder and Humbolt.

Feenstra Kuiper, J. 1921. *Japan en de Buitenwereld in de Achttiende Eeuw.* The Hague: Martinus Nijhoff.

Fitzgerald, C. P. 1961. *China: A short cultural history.* 3d ed. London: The Cresset Press.

Flexner, Abraham. 1925. *Medical education: A comparative study.* New York: Macmillan Co.

Flexner, Simon, and Flexner, James Thomas. 1941. *William Henry Welch and the heroic age of American medicine.* New York: The Viking Press.

Frois, Luis. 1955. Das Doencas, Medicos E Mezinhas. *Kulturgegensatze Europa-Japan (1585),* sec. 9, pp. 206–11. Translated by J. F. Schutte, S.J. Tokyo: Sophia Universität.

Fujikawa Yū. 1911. *Geschichter der medizin in Japan.* Tokyo: Kaiserlich-Japanisches Unterrichtsministerium.

Fukaura Jisaburō. 1915. Rampō Igaku no Sōjutsuka Narabayashike. *Rekishi Chiri* 26, no. 4: 69–73.

Fukushima Gentō. 1967. Higeki no rangakusha, Takano Chōei. *Igaku no Ayumi* 60, no. 3: 155–58.

Fukuzawa Yukichi. 1960. *The autobiography of Fukuzawa Yukichi.* Translated by Eikichi Kiyooka. Tokyo: Hokuseidō.

Gardner, K. B. 1962. Engelbert Kaempfer's Japanese library. *Asia Major*, n.s., no. 7, pts. 1–2: 74–78.

Garrison, Fielding H. 1929. *An introduction to the history of medicine: With medical chronology, suggestions for study, and biographical data.* 4th ed. Philadelphia and London: Saunders.

Golownin, V. M. 1821. *Narrative of my captivity in Japan.* London: Henry Colburn and Co.

———. 1953. *Japan and the Japanese: Captain Golownin.* New and revised edition. 2 vols. London.

Goodman, Grant Kohn. 1967. *The Dutch impact on Japan (1640–1853).* Leiden: E. J. Brill.

Gowen, Herbert H. 1928. *A precursor of Perry or the story of Takano Nagahide.* Seattle: University of Washington Press.

Gragg, William F. 1860. *A cruise in the U.S. Steam Frigate, Mississippi, Wm. C. Nicholson, Captain, to China and Japan, from July 1857 to February 1860.* Boston.

Gray, Basil. 1953. Sloane and the Kaempfer collections. *British Museum Quarterly* 18: 20–23.

Greene, D. C. 1907. Correspondence between William II of Holland and the Shogun of Japan, A.D. 1844. *Transactions of the Asiatic Society of Japan* 24, pt. 4: 99–123.

Griffis, William Elliott. 1877. *The Mikado's empire.* New York: Harper and Bros.

———. 1901. *Verbeck of Japan, a citizen of no country: A life story of foundation work inaugurated by Guido Fridolin Verbeck.* New York: Revell Co.

Guiart, J. 1947. *Histoire de la médecine Française.* Lyons.

Guillier, O. 1882. *Histoire de L'Hôpital Notre-Dame de Pitié, 1618–1882.* Paris.

Gurlt, E., Wernich, A., and Hirsch, August. 1932. *Biographisches Lexikon der hervorragenden Ärzte aller Zeiten und Völker.* 2d ed. by W. Haberling, H. Vierordt, and F. Hübotter. Berlin and Vienna: Urban & Schwarzenberg.

Guzman, Luis de. 1601. *Historia de las missiones que han hecho los religiosos de la Compañía de Iesus, para predicar El Sancto Euangelio en la India Oriental, y en los Reynos de la China y Iapon.* Alacalá.

Halbertsma, K. T. A. 1941–42. Beteekenis van de Hollandsche Geneeskunde voor Japan in Haar Historische Ontwikkeling. *Bijdragen tot de Geschiedenis der Geneeskunde* 21, nos. 1–6.

Hasama, B. 1933. Geschichtiche Daten über die Ersteinfuhsung des Deutschen Medizin al wesens in Japan. *Südhoffs Archiv für Geschichte der Medizin* 26: 329–39.

Hawks, Francis L. 1856. *Narrative of the expedition of an American squadron to the China seas and Japan.* Washington, D.C.: Beverly Tucker, Senate Printer.

Hearn, Lafcadio. 1917. *Life and literature.* Selected and edited with an introduction by John Erskine. New York: Dodd, Mead & Co.

Hoyanagi Matsumi. 1967. Re-appreciation of Inō's Maps, the first maps of Japan based on actual survey. *Geographical Reports of Tokyo Metropolitan University*, no. 2.

Huard, P., and Huang, Kuang-Ming (M. Wong). 1959. *La Médecine Chinoise au Cours des Siècles.* Paris: Dacosta.

Hübotter, F. 1929. *Die Chinesische Medizin zu Beginn des XX. Jahrhunderts, und ihr historischer Entwicklungsang* (China Library on Asia Major, 1). Leipzig: Schindler.

Hyma, Albert. 1942. *The Dutch in the Far East.* Ann Arbor, Mich.: George Wahr.

Instituto de Alta Cultura. 1598. Cartos que os padres e irmaos da Companhia de Jesus escreuerai dos reynos de Japão et China. . . . 1549–1589. *Jesuit letters from missions (the East)*, vol. 1. Lisbon: Evora.

Itazawa Takeo. 1955. *Nichiran bunka kōshōshi no kenkyū.* Tokyo: Yoshikawa kobunkan.

———. 1960. *Shiboruto*, pp. 75–76. Tokyo: Yoshikawa kobunkan.

Kaempfer, Engelbert. 1694. "Dissertatio medica inauguralis sistens decadem observationum exoticarum: I. De Agno Scytica, seu fructu Borometz; II. De Amaritie Caspii Maris; III. De Mumia Nativa Persica; IV. De Torpedine Sinus Persici; V. De Dfjerenang, id est, Sanguine Draconis, ex fructibus Palma Conifera spinosa elicito; VI. De Dracunculo Persarum; VII. De Andrum, endemia Malabarorum Hydrocele; VIII. De Perical, indigena Malabaris Hypersarcosi ulcerose Pedum; IX. De Curatione Colicae per Acupuncturam, Japonensibus usitata; X. De Moxa, Materia Cauteriorum apud Chinenses Japoniosque usitata." Doctoral dissertation, University of Leiden.

———. 1712. *Amoenitatum Exoticarum Politico-Physico-Medicarum Fasciculi V, Quibus continentur Variae Relationes, Observationes & Descriptiones Rerum Persicarum & Ulterioris Asiae.* Lemgo: Meyeri.

———. 1727. *The history of Japan.* Translated by J. G. Scheuchzer. 2 vols. London. (a) *Histoire naturelle, civile, et ecclesiastique de l'Empire du Japon.* 2 vols. La Haye, 1729. *Ibid.* 3 vols. Amsterdam, 1732. (b) *De Beschryving van Japan-Uyt het oorspronkelyk Hoog Duytsch.*

Manuscript by J. G. Scheuchzer. Translated from English into Dutch. Amsterdam, 1733. (c) *Geschichte und Beschreibung von Japan: Aus den Originalhandschriften* . . . . Edited by Christian Wilhelm Dohn. 2 vols. Lemgo: Im Verlage der Meyerschen Buchhandlung, 1777–79.

Kaempfer, Engelbert (1651–1716), Philipp Franz von Siebold (1796–1866): Gedenkschrift: Erganzt durch eine Darstellung der deutschen Japanologie: Deutsch und Japanisch. 1966. *Deutsche Gesellschaft für Natur- und Völkerkunde Ostasiens* 28.

Kattendyke, W. J. C. 1924. *Un Mission Au Japon, Le Japon en 1857, Extraits Du Journal Du Chevalier W. J. C. Huyssen de Kattendyke.* Paris: Fischbacher.

Keene, Donald. 1952. *The Japanese discovery of Europe: Honda Toshiaki and other discoverers, 1720–1798.* London: Routledge & Kegan Paul.

Kleiweg de Zwaan, J. P. 1917. *Völkerkundliches und Geschichtliches über die Heilkunde der Chinesen ünd Japaner mit Besonderer Berücksichtigung Holländischer Einflüsse.* Haarlem: De Erven Loosjes.

Körner, Hans. 1967. Siebold: Beitrage zur Familiengeschichte: Bearbeitet in Auftrage von Friederich-Karl von Siebold. *Die Würzburger Siebold: Eine Gelehrtenfamilie des 18 und 19 Jahrhunderts,* pt. 1, no. 3. Archives of German Families, vols. 34–35. Neustadt on the Aisch: Degener and Co.

Krieger, C. C. 1940. *The infiltration of European civilization in Japan during the 18th century.* Leiden: E. J. Brill.

Krusenstern, Adam Johann von. 1810–12. *Reise um die Welt in den Jahren 1803, 1804, 1805 und 1806, auf Befehl seiner kaiserlichen Majestät Alexander des Ersten auf den Schiffen Nadeshda und Neva unter den Commando des Capitains von der kaiserlichen Marine A. J. von Krusenstern.* St. Petersburg: Gedruckt in der Schnoorschen Buchdruckerei.

————. 1814. *Atlas zur Reise um die Welt unternommen auf Befehl seiner kaiserlichen Majestät Alexander des ersten auf den Schiffen Nadeshda und Neva. unter dem Commando des Capitains von Krusenstern.* St. Petersburg. Translated by R. B. Hoppner. 2 vols. London: John Murray, 1813; Paris, 1821.

Kure Shūzō. 1896. *Shiboruto.* Tokyo: Eirandō; Tōhōdō shoten.

————. 1914. *Mitsukuri Gempō.* Tokyo: Dai Nihon Tosho Kabushiki Kaisha.

————. 1926. *Shiburuto sensei sono shōgai oyobi kōgyo.* Tokyo: Tōhōdō shoten.

————. 1933. *Einfluss der fremden, insbesondere der Deutschen Medizin auf der Japanische, 1700–1933.* Tokyo: Jubilaumsband der O.A.G.

Lauer, Hans H. 1966. Zwei mutige Frauen in ihrer Zeit: Josepha von Siebold und ihre Tochter Charlotte Heidenreich-von Siebold. *Med. Monatsspiegel* 2.

Leers, Johann v. 1942. Der Japan-Siebold die Groszleistung eines deutschen Ärztes. *Deutsche Medizinische Wochenschrift* 68, no. 47: 1151–53.

Lensen, George Alexander. 1955. *Russia's Japan Expedition of 1852–1855*. Gainesville: University of Florida Press.

Lindroth, Sten, ed. 1952. C. P. Thunberg, by Nils Svedelius. *Swedish men of science*. Translated by Burnett Anderson. Stockholm.

Loewenson, Leo. 1935–36. Russian documents in the British Museum, II. Seventeenth century: The manuscripts of Engelbert Kaempfer. *Slavonic Rev.* 14: 661–69.

Ma Eikoh. 1959. Japan's encounter with Western medical science. *Bulletin of the History of Medicine* 33, no. 4: 315–29.

———. 1961. The impact of Western medicine in Japan: Memoirs of a pioneer, Sugita Gempaku, 1733–1817. *Archives Internationales d'histoire des sciences* 14, nos. 54–55: 65–84.

Magnus-Levy, Adolf. 1944. The heroic age of German medicine. *Bulletin of the History of Medicine* 16: 331–42.

Mann, F. 1962. *Acupuncture: The ancient Chinese art of healing*. London: William Heinemann.

Masselman, George. 1963. *The cradle of colonialism*. New Haven and London: Yale University Press.

Meier-Lemgo, Karl. 1937. *Engelbert Kaempfer, der erste deutsche Forschungsreisende 1651–1716: Leben, reisen nach den bisher unveröffentlichten handschriften Kaempfers im Britischen Museum bearbeitet.* 28 plates. Stuttgart: Strecker & Schroder.

———. 1952. Das Stammbuch Engelbert Kaempfers. *Mitt. lipp. Gesch.* 21.

———. 1960. *Engelbert Kaempfer, erforscht das seltsame Asien*. Hamburg: Cram, de Gruyter & Co.

———. 1962. *Geschichte der Stadt Lemgo*. Lemgo: F. L. Wagener.

———. 1965a. Die Briefe Engelbert Kaempfers. *Akademie der wissenschaften und der literatur: Abhandlungen der mathematisch-naturwissenschaftlichen klasse*, no. 6. Wiesbaden: Franz Steiner.

———. 1965b. Die wirkung und geltung Engelbert Kaempfers bei der nachwelt. *Sonderdruck Lippische Mitteilungen aus Geschichte und Landeskunde* 34.

———. 1968. *Die Reisetagebücher Engelbert Kaempfers*. Weisbaden: Franz Steiner Verlag GmbH.

Mestler, Gordon E. 1954–57. A galaxy of old Japanese medical books with miscellaneous notes on early medicine in Japan. *Bulletin of the*

Medical Library Association 42, pt. 1, no. 3; 42, pt. 2, no. 4; 44, pt. 3, no. 2; 44, pt. 4, no. 3; 45, no. 2.

————. 1957. Introduction to Western influences in pre-Meiji Japanese medicine. *Proceedings of the Royal Society of Medicine* 50, no. 12: 1005–13.

Mitsukuri D. 1877. The early study of Dutch in Japan. *Transactions of the Asiatic Society of Japan* 5, pt. 1: 207–16.

Molhuysen P. C., and Kossmann, Fr. K. H. 1933. *Nieuw Nederlandsch Biografisch Woordenboek*. Leiden: A. W. Sijthoff.

Montanus, Arnoldus. 1670. *Atlas Japonesis*. London: John Ogilby.

————. 1680. *Ambassades Memorables de la Compagnie des Indes Orientales des Provinces Unies vers les Empereurs du Japon*. Amsterdam: Jacob de Meurs.

Mori Kōichi, trans. 1942. Rangaku Kotohajime [Die Anfrange der Holland-Kunde]. *Monumenta Nipponica* 5, no. 1: 144–66 and no. 2: 215–36.

Morison, Samuel Eliot. 1967. *"Old Bruin" Commodore Matthew C. Perry, 1794–1858*. Boston and Toronto: Little, Brown & Co.

Morse, William R. 1934. *Chinese medicine*. New York: Hoeber.

Murdoch, James. 1926. *A history of Japan*. vol. 3. Revised and edited by Joseph H. Longford. London: Kegan Paul, Trench, Trubner and Co.

Murdoch, James, and Yamagata, I. 1949. *A history of Japan*, vol. 2. Third impression. London: Routledge & Kegan Paul.

Museum of Natural History. *Plantae ab Engelberto Kempfero in Belgio praecipue HORTO LUGDANO BATAVO collectae*. London.

————. *Volumen Plantarum in Japonia collectarum ab. Engelberto Kempfero M.D. annis 1691 et 1692, Additae subfinem Plantae aliquot ab eodem in Persia et Insula Ceylon repertae*. London.

Nachod, O. 1897. *Die Beziehungen der Niederlandischen Ostindischen Kompagnie zu Japan im Siebzehnten Jahrhundert*. Leipzig: Friese.

Nagasaki Art Association. 1965. *Dejima Oranda-yashiki no Kei*. Nagasaki.

Nagasaki Prefectural Library. Letters from P. F. von Siebold to his daughter Ine. Nagasaki.

Nagasaki Shiyakusho, ed. 1926. *Nagasaki to kaigai bunka*. Nagasaki.

————. 1961. *Nagasaki Daigaku Igakubu, Nagasaki Igaku Hyakunenshi*. Nagasaki.

Nagayo Sensai. 1800. *Shōkō Shishi*. Tokyo: Tōhōdō shoten.

Nakamura Takeshi. 1965. The contribution of foreigners. From "The importation of Western science during the Tokugawa period." *Journal of World History* 9, no. 2: 294–319.

Naumann, Moritz. 1868. *Chronik des Bonner Freundeskränzchens: Den Mitgliedern des Kränzchens zum 25—jahrigen Jubiläum gewidmet*, p. 79. Bonn: Carl Georgi.

Needham, Joseph. 1956. *Science and civilization in China: History of scientific thought*, vol. 2. Cambridge.

———. 1967. The roles of Europe and China in the evolution of oecumenical science. *Journal of Asian History* 1, pt. 1: 3–32.

Needham, J., and Lu, Gwei-Djen. Contributions to the 1966 Wellcome Symposium on Medicine and Culture. Paper read at Wellcome Symposium, September 28, 1966, at Wellcome Museum, London.

Nishi Seiho. 1960. Waga kuni shoki no kaibō. *Nippon Iji Shimpō*, no. 186: 57–60.

Nordenskjold, Erik. 1935. *The history of biology*. New York: Alfred A. Knopf.

Numata Jirō. 1937. Ran'i Pompe. *Rekishi Chiri* 70, no. 2: 137–47.

———. 1950. *Bakumatsu Yōgakushi*. Tokyo: Tōkōshoin.

———. 1961. *Yōgaku denrai no Rekishi*. Tokyo: Shibundō.

———. 1966. *Bakumatsu ni Okeru Ranjin Kyōshi Pompe no Jiseki*. Tokyo.

Ogata Kōan. 1858. *Choreri Chi Jun*. n.p.

Ogawa Teizō. 1962. Oranda Shōgatsu no Hitobito. *Nippon Iji Shimpō*, no. 21: 12–14.

———. 1963a. Juntendō no Rekishi. Juntendō Sōritsu 125 Shūnen Kinen Kōen.

———. 1963b. Nippon no igakushi kara, no. 6: Siebold no Shōgai. *Nippon Iji Shimpō*, nos. 22, 23, and 24.

———. 1964–65. Satō Taizen Den. *Juntendō Igaku* 10, no. 1: 53–58; 10, no. 2: 119–23; 10, no. 3: 211–13; 10, no. 4: 76–80; 11, no. 1: 40–44; 11, no. 3: 185–87.

Ōtori Ranzaburō. 1962. Rankan nisshi no ishigakuteki kenkyū. *Nihon ishigaku zasshi* 20.

Ōtsuki Gentaku. 1788a. *Rangaku Kaitei*. 2 vols. n.p.

———. 1788b. *Ransetsu Benwaku*. Edo.

———. 1826. *Jūtei Kaitai Shinsho*. 6 vols. Edo.

Ōtsuki Shigeo. 1912. *Bansui Zonkyō*. Tokyo.

Paske-Smith, M. 1930. *Western barbarians in Japan and Formosa in Tokugawa days, 1603–1868*. Kobe: J. L. Thompson.

Pompe van Meerdervoort, J. L. C. 1859. On the study of natural sciences in Japan. *Journal of the North China Branch of the Royal Asiatic Society of Great Britain and Ireland* 1: 211–221.

———. 1860. Dissection of a Japanese criminal. *Journal of North China Branch of the Royal Asiatic Society of Great Britain and Ireland* 2: 85–91.

———. 1867–68. *Vijf Jaren in Japan (1857–186–): Bijdragen tot De Kennis Van Het Japanische Keizerrijk En Zijne Bevolking*. Leiden: Firma Van Den Heuvell and Van Santen.

Prestage, Edgar. 1933. *The Portuguese pioneers*. London: A. and C. Black.

Rangaku Shiryō Kenkyūkai, comp. 1954. *Yōgaku Kotohajime Ten.* Tokyo.

Ray, John. 1848. *Correspondence of John Ray.* Edited by Edward Lankester, Ray Society. London: C. and J. Adland.

Read, Bernard E. 1931. Chinese materia medica—animal drugs. *Peking Natural History Bulletin* 5, pt. 4: 37–80, and 6, pt. 1: 1–102.

Reinhardt, W. 1962. Yamawaki Tōyō. *Itan.* 25: 17.

Reischauer, Edwin Oldfather. 1946. *Japan, past and present.* New York: Alfred A. Knopf.

———. 1952. *Japan.* New York: Alfred A. Knopf.

Ricci, Matthew. 1953. *China in the sixteenth century: The journals of Matthew Ricci, 1583–1610.* Translated by Louis J. Gallagher, S.J. New York: Random House.

Rômer, L. S. A. M. von. 1921. *Historische Schetsen: Een Inleiding Tot Het Vierde Congres Der Far Eastern Association of Tropical Medicine.* Batavia: Javasche Boekhandel en Drukkerij.

Rowbotham, Arnold H. 1966. *Missionary and mandarin: The Jesuits at the court of China.* New York: Russell & Russell.

Rundall, Thomas, ed. 1850. *Memorials of the Empire of Japon in the XVI and XVII centuries.* London: Hakluyt Society.

Sacadura, S. da Costa, and Machado, J. T. Montalvão. 1965. Andanças do ensina médico na capital (Do Hospital Real de Todos-os-Santos ao Hospital de Santa Maria). *Médico (Porto)* 34: 140–73.

St. John, James Augustus. 1831. *Lives of celebrated travellers.* London.

St. John Brooks, E. 1954. *Sir Hans Sloane.* London: Batchworth Press.

Sansom, George B. 1952. *Japan: A short cultural history.* Rev. ed. London: The Cresset Press.

———. 1962. *The Western world and Japan.* 2d ed. New York: Alfred A. Knopf.

———. 1963. *A history of Japan, 1615–1867.* Stanford: Stanford University Press.

Schilling, Dorotheus, O.F.M. 1937. *Os Portuguéses e a introdução da medicine no Japão.* Coimbra.

Schilling, Dorotheus P. 1949. Wohltäter der Hospitaler St. Joseph und St. Anna der Franziskaner in Miyako (1594–1597). *Neue Zeitschrift für Missionswissenschaft* 1.

Schilling, Konrad. 1931. *Das Schulwesen der Jesuiten in Japan, 1551–1614.* Münster.

Schmid, Günther. 1942. Über Ph. Fr. v. Siebolds Reise Nach Japan. *Botanisches Archiv.* 43: 487–530.

Schöffer, Ivo. 1936. *A short history of The Netherlands.* Amsterdam: Allert de Lange.

Schoute, D. 1929. *De Geneeskunde in den Dienst der Oost-Indische Compagnie in Nederlandsch-Indie.* Amsterdam: J. H. DeBussy.

Science Council of Japan and Botanical Society of Japan. 1953. *Forskningsmaterial rorende C. P. Thunberg.* Tokyo.

Sekiuma Fujihiko. 1938. *Seiigaku Tōzen Shiwa.* Tokyo: Tōhōdō shoten.

Sencourt, Robert. 1933. *Napoleon III: The modern emperor.* New York: D. Appleton-Century Co.

Serrurier, L. 1896. *Bibliothèque Japonaise, Catalogue Raisonné des Livres et des Manuscrits Japonais.* Leiden: E. J. Brill.

Shiiboruto Sensei Torai Hyakunen Kinenkai. 1924. *Shiiboruto Sensei Torai Hyakunen Kinen Rombunshū.* Nagasaki.

Siebold, Alexander von. 1901. *Japan's accession to the community of nations.* Translated from the German with an introduction by Charles Lowe. London: Kegan Paul, Trench, Trubner and Co.

———. 1903. *Philipp Franz von Siebolds letzte Reise nach Japan, 1859 bis 1862.* Berlin: von Kisak Tamai.

Siebold, P. F. von. *Overzicht van de Geschiedenis van het Rijksmuseum voor Völkerkunde, 1837–1937.* Leiden.

———. 1824. *De Historia Naturalis in Japonia statu.* Batavia.

———. 1852. *Geschichte der Entdeckungen in Seegebiet von Japan nebst Erklarung des Atlas von Land und Seekarten vom Japanischen Reiche und dessen neben und Schutzlandern.* Leiden.

———. 1854. *Urkundliche Darstellung der Bestrebungen von Niederland und Russland zur Eröffnung Japan's für Die Schiff fahrt und den Seehandel aller Nationen,* pp. 1–34. Bonn: beim Verfasser.

———. 1862. *Catalogue de la Bibliothèque apportée au Japon.* Deshima: Niederlandische Druckerei.

———. 1896. Nekrolog zu seiner hundertjahrisen Gebutstagsfeier. Compiled by Hans Körner. *Der Ostasiatische Lloyd* 10.

———. 1897. *Nippon: Archiv zur Beschreibung von Japan und dessen Nebe- nund Schutzlandern Jezo mit den südlichen Kurilen, Sachalin, Korea und den Liukiu-Inseln.* Presented by his sons, Alexander and Heinrich Freiherren von Siebold. Vol. 8 (with 47 illus.), vol. 36 (with 53 illus. and 1 map), and *Nippon,* an archive of descriptions of Japan, complete from Siebold's first work in Japan, 1823–30. Würzburg and Leipzig: Leo Woerl.

Siebold, P. F. B. von, Temminck, C. J., Schlegel, H., and de Haan, W. 1833. *Fauna Japonica.* 5 vols. Leiden: Verfasser.

Siebold, P. F. B. von, and Zuccarini, J. G. 1835–41. *Flora Japonica.* Leiden: Verfasser; Amsterdam: J. Muller; Leipzig: L. Voss; Paris: L. Roret; St. Petersburg: J. Brieff; Vienna: Schaumburg.

Siebold, Werner. 1943. *Ein Deutscher Gewinnt Japans Herz*. Leipzig: von Hase und Koehler.

Singer, Charles, and Underwood, E. Ashworth. 1962. *A short history of medicine*. 2d ed. Oxford: Clarendon Press.

Sloane, Sir Hans. 1707 and 1725. *A voyage to the islands of Madeira, Barbados, Nieves, St. Christopher's and Jamaica*. 2 vols. London.

———. 1725. Archives at the British Museum, no. 4048, f. 92, 93.

———. 1753. *Authentic copies of the codicils belonging to the last will and testament of Sir Hans Sloane, bart. deceased, which relates to his collection of books, and curiosities*. London: Daniel Browne.

Smith, G. 1861. *Ten weeks in Japan*. London: Longman, Green, Longman, and Roberts.

Steenis-Kruseman, M. J. 1950. Malaysian plant collectors and collections. In *Flora Malesiana*, vol. 1. Edited by C. G. G. J. Van Steenis. Djakarta.

Stephen, Sir Leslie, and Lee, Sir Sidney, eds. *The dictionary of national biography*, s.v. "Sloane, Sir Hans." England.

Steudel, Johannes. 1942. Deutsche Ärzte in Japan als Mittler der Abendlaendischen Medizin. *Med. Welt*. 16: 1138–41.

———. 1960. *Die Siebolds: ein Hervorragendes Ärzte-Geschlecht aus dem Dürener Lande*. Düren: Rhld. Degen and Kuth.

Sticker, G. 1927. K. K. von Siebold. *Festschrift zum 46, Deutschen Ärztetag im Würzburg*. Würzburg.

Stromberg, Andrew. 1931. *A history of Sweden*. New York: Macmillan Co.

Sugita Gempaku. 1795. *Oranda Iji Mondō*. 2 vols. Edo.

———. 1810. *Keiei Yawa*. Edo.

———. 1942. Rangaku Kotohajime. Translated by K. Mori. *Monumenta Nipponica* 5, no. 1: 144–66 and no. 2: 215–36.

———. 1959. *Rangaku Kotohajime*. Edited by Ogata Tomio. Tokyo: Kōgakusha.

Suzuki Y. 1933. *Rangaku zenseijidai to ranchū no shōgai*. Tokyo: Iji Shinshikyoku.

Svedelius, Nils. 1944a. Carl Peter Thunberg (1743–1828): On his Bicentury. *Isis* 35, pt. 2: 128–34.

———. 1944b. Carl Peter Thunberg (1743–1828). *Sartryck ur Svenska Linne-Sallskapets Arsskrift* 27.

Taniguchi M. and Bowers, J. Z. 1965. Pompe van Meerdervoort and the first Western medical school in Japan. *Journal Med. Ed*. 40: 448–54.

Tanizaki Junichiro. 1957. *The Makioka sisters*. New York: Alfred A. Knopf.

Ten Kate, H. 1901. Erinnerungen an Philipp Franz von Siebold. *Mittheilungen der Deutschen Gesellschaft für Natur- und Völkerkunde Ostasiens* 9: 1–6.

Ten Rhijne, Willem. 1669 and 1672. *Meditationes, In Magni Hippocratis Textum XXIV. de Vet Med.* Leiden.

————. 1683 and 1690. *Dissertatio de arthritide: Mantissa schematica de acupunctura et orationes tres de chymiae et botanices antiquate et dignitate, de physiognomia et de monstris.* London, The Hague, and Leipzig.

————. 1686. Schediasma de Promontorio Bonaespei; ejusve tractus incolis Hottentottis, accurante, brevusque notas addente Henr. Screta S. a Zavoriziz. *Ampliss. Soc. Indiae Or. Medici. & a consiliis Justitae.* Meisteri: Scafusii Impensis Joh. Mart.

————. 1687. *Verhandelinge Van de Asiatise Melaatsheid na een naaukeuriger ondersoek ten dienste van het gemeen.* Amsterdam: Abraham von Someren.

The acceptance of Western culture in Japan. 1964. *Monumenta Nipponica* 9, nos. 3–4: 1–85.

The Harley Street Calendar. 1929. London: H. H. Bashford.

Thomson, W. W. 1938. Some aspects of the life and times of Sir Hans Sloane. *Ulster Medical Journal* 7: 4–5.

Thunberg, C. P. Thunbergiana, vols. 1–14: Testimonia & Diplomata; Biographica; Orationes, etc.; Fauna Capensis, Ornithologia, etc.; Amphibiolog., Icht., & Entomol; Botanica, Animalia & Vegetabilia in Sacr. Ser.; Diaeta, Materia Medica, etc.; Donatio Animalium; Donatio Herbarii; Bibliotheca; Zoologica; Entomologia. Uppsala, Sweden: Archives of the University Library.

————. 1794. *Icones Plantarum Japonicarum: Quas in Insulis Japonicis Annus 1775 et 1776 Collegit et Descripsit.* Uppsala: Johann Fred Edman.

————. 1795–96. A voyage to the southern parts of Europe and to the Cape of Good Hope . . . 1770–1773. Two expeditions to the interior part of the country adjacent to the Cape of Good Hope, and a voyage to the island of Java . . . 1773–1775. A voyage to Japan and travels in different parts of that Empire . . . 1775–1776. Travels in the Empire of Japan, and in the islands of Java and Ceylon, together with the voyage home. *Travels in Europe, Africa and Asia, made between the years 1770 and 1779,* vols. 1, 2, 3, and 4. 3d ed. London: Rivington.

Thunberg, C. P., Winberg, L., and Widmark, F. r. 01. 1825. Thesis: *Florula Javanica,* pts. 1–2. Uppsala.

Titsingh, Isaak. 1785–91. *Zes en veertig ergenhandlige brieven aan de Heer Titsingh, geschreven door Sige-Senoski, Nakagawa-Sjunnan, Ko-zack.* Fol. H. Archives of Kyoto University Library, Kyoto.

————. 1822. *Illustrations of Japan.* Translated from the French by F. Shoberl. London.

Trautz, F. M. 1937. Kaempfer und Siebold. *Deutsche Akademie Muenchen Mitteilungen* 12: 1–10.

Tuge Hideomi. 1961. *Historical development of science and technology in Japan.* Tokyo: Kokusai Bunka Shinkōkai.

Ueno Masuzo. 1964. The Western influence on natural history in Japan. *Monumenta Nipponica* 19, nos. 3–4: 81–105.

Vallery-Radot, R. 1920. *The life of Pasteur.* Translated from the French by R. L. Devonshire. New York.

van Reede tot Drakestein, H. A. 1682. Preface to *Hortus Malabaricus.* Amsterdam.

Veith, Ilza. 1949. *Huang Ti Nei Ching Su Wen: The yellow emperor's classic of internal medicine.* Baltimore: Williams & Wilkins.

———. 1950. Medicine in Japan. *Ciba Symposia* 11, no. 4.

von Moll, C. E. 1822. *Mittheilung aus seinem Briefwechsel,* pp. 852ff. 3 vols. Heidingsfeld (Augsburg, 1834).

von Wagenseil, F. 1959. Die Drei Ersten unter Europaeischem (Hollaendischem) Einfluss Entstandenem Japanischen Anatomiebuecher. *Sudhoff Archiv Ges. Med.* 43: 61–85.

Wada Shinjiro. 1941. *Nakagawa Junan sensei.* Kyoto: Ritsumei-kan Shippanbu.

Wagner, Moriz. 1866. Zur Erinnerung an Philip Franz V. Siebold. *Beilage zur Allgemeinen Zeitung* 317.

Wallnofer, H., and von Rottauscher, A. 1965. *Chinese folk medicine.* Translated by Marion Palmeda. New York: Crown Publishers.

Walworth, Arthur. 1946. *Black ships off Japan.* New York: A. A. Knopf.

Wap, D. 1859. *De Stad Utrecht: Rijks-Kweekschool Voor Militaire Geneeskundigen en Rijks-Hospital, -Voorheen Het Duitsche Huis.* Utrecht: Broese.

Warner, Oliver. 1965. *The sea and the sword, the Baltic, 1630–1945.* New York: William Morrow and Co.

Washington, D.C. National Archives. Record Group 59. Diplomatic Dispatches Netherlands, vol. 14: Folsom to Secretary Webster, June 26, 1850–October 14, 1853.

Whitney, Willis Norton. 1885. Notes on the history of medical progress in Japan. *Transactions of the Asiatic Society of Japan* 12: 245–399.

Willman, Oloff Erichson. 1667. The journal of the voyages of Nils Matson into Asia and Africa. *A voyage to the East Indies, together with a short account of the kingdom of Japan and its emperor.* Wussingsborgh, Sweden.

Wong, K. Chi Min, and Wu, Lien-Teh. 1934. *History of Chinese medicine: Being a chronicle of medical happenings in China from ancient times to the present period.* Tientsin: Tientsin Press.

Wooley, W. A. 1881. Historical notes on Nagasaki. *Transactions of the Asiatic Society of Japan* 9: 125–51.

Yabuti Kiyosi. 1965. The pre-history of modern science in Japan. From "The importation of Western science during the Tokugawa period." *Journal of World History* 9, no. 2: 208–32.

Yamazaki Tasuku. 1958. *Nagayo Sensai Shōkō Shishi*. Tokyo: Ishiyaku Shuppan Co. (Nihon Ishi Gakkai, ed. *Igaku kotenshū*, vol. 2).

———. 1961a. Matsumoto Ryōjun. *Nagasaki Daigaku Igakubu: Nagasaki Igaku Hyakunenshi*. Nagasaki.

———. 1961b. Pompe van Meerdervoort. *Nagasaki Daigaku Igakubu: Nagasaki Igaku Hyakunenshi*. Nagasaki.

Yanaga Chitoshi. 1960. *Japan since Perry*. Hamden, Conn.: Archon Books.

Zoku-Tsūshin zenran, Ranjin Shīboruto chōkō ikken. Tokyo: Kure Collection, Medical Library, Tokyo University.

Note: The author is currently working on a book on Chinese medicine based on the Peking Union Medical College.

Index

Acupuncture: basis for use of, 5; described by Ten Rhijne, 35; indications for use of, 7; as treatment for *senki*, 80

Alexander II, czar of Russia, 132

Alexander VI, Pope: and Treaty of Tordesillas, 14–15

Almeida, Luis de: first to practice Western medicine in Japan, 11–13; and trade with Japanese, 12–13

Anatomia publica, 64

Anatomy. *See* Dissection

Aoki Konyō, 62–63, 67, 101

Arai Hakuseki, 61

Bakufu: attitude toward Siebold upon his second visit, 162–66; outlawed all Western studies except medicine, 142–43; sponsored medical schools for *Kampō*, 92–93

Batavia: headquarters of Dutch Asian empire, 17

Bauduin, Antonius F., Dr.: successor to Pompe van Meerdervoort, 192

Blasquez, Petrus Baptista, Brother: established Franciscan hospital in Japan, 15–16

Botany: introduced to Japan by Thunberg, 73

Boym, Michael, 37

British Museum: founded, 56; Kaempfer collection at, 56–57

Buddhism: importance to Japanese medicine, 5–6; mentioned, 4, 8, 47–48

Burger, Heinrich, 116

Burmann, Nikolas: patron and friend of Thunberg, 75, 79, 86

Busch, Daniel, 31

Cadaver. *See* Dissection

Camphuijs, Johannes, 36, 46

Cape Colony: Thunberg's botanical studies of, 77, 86, 88

Capellen, Baron van der: commissioned Siebold as physician to Deshima, 108, 110

Charles XI, king of Spain, 42

China: influence on Japanese culture, 3–9

Cholera: epidemic of 1858, 186–88

Chung-i: basis of belief in, 4; diagnostic approaches of, 5; introduced to Japan, 3; therapeutic techniques of, 5

Cleyer, Andreas, 37, 46

239

mens, 111; married Kusumoto Taki (O-taki-san), 115; year's confinement, 124, 125
— life in exile: constructed classical Japanese garden at Lagan Rijndik, Leiderdorp, 131–32; established National Ethnographic Museum at Leiden, 133–34
— second visit to Japan, 160–66; as adviser on foreign relations, 162–65

Sloane, Sir Hans, 54–56

Smallpox: epidemic, first official record of, 7; Siebold's observations on, 118
— vaccination: introduced by Otto Mohnike, 195; Japanese attitudes during Siebold's tenure, 110; used by Satō Taizen, 142

Society of Jesus: D'Almeida as missionary of, 11, 13

Spain: and conflict with Portugal over missionary rights in Japan, 14–15

Steigerthal, George, Dr., 55

Steuler, Willem der: antagonism toward Siebold, 122–26; arrival with Siebold at Deshima, 103, 108–9

Sugawara Michizane, 69

Sugita Gempaku, 67–71; description of dissection, 70; importance to *Rangaku*, 150; studied Western medicine, 67–68, 70; teacher of Ōtsuki Gentaku, 93–94; translated *Tafel Anatomia*, 70–72; mentioned, 92, 95, 201

Sylvius, Franciscus (Franz de la Böe): teacher of Ten Rhijne, 32

Tafel Anatomia: translated into Japanese (*Kaitai Shinsho*), 70–72

Taihō Code of Laws, 6

Takahashi Sakusaemon (Kageyasu): court astronomer, 121–22

Takano Chōei: advocated opening of Japanese ports to the West, 128; life of, 126–29; published *Igen suyō*, 127; student of Siebold, 126; mentioned, 130, 142, 201

Takebe Seian, 93

Takeuchi Gendō, 129, 162

Takeya Ryōtei, 182, 183

Tamba Yasuyori: author of *Ishinho*, 7

T'ang dynasty, 3–4

Tao: in explanation of *Chung-i*, 4

Tashiro Sanki (Dodo): introduced *Ri-shu* school to Japan, 8; mentioned, 65

Tea plant: Ten Rhijne's studies of, 36

Tekiteki-sai Juku: founded, 94, 143–48

Ten Rhijne, Willem, **31–38**; childhood and education, 32–33; described Chinese and Japanese medicine to West, 35; described tea plant to West, 36; travels to Japan, 33–36; mentioned, 26

Thunberg, Carl Pieter, **72–90**; agreed to collect specimens for Nikolas Burmann, 75; Cape Colony expedition, 77; on *hofreis* to Edo, 81–85; importance to West, 200–201; published *Fauna Japonica*, *Flora Japonica*, and *Florula Javanica*, 87; return trip to Sweden, 85–86; student of Carolus Linnaeus, 73–75, 88–90 *passim;* studied medicine and surgery in Paris, 75–76; visited Batavia, 77; mentioned, 2, 26, 100

Tokugawa shogunate, 48, 60–62 *passim*
— Iemitsu: banned Jesuit religious and scientific books, 24–25; closed Japan to the West, 19
— Ieyasu: persecution of Christian missionaries, 17
— Tsunayoshi, 48
— Yoshimune: contributions to rise of Western medicine in Japan, 61–62; programs for Japan, 61, 62

Tordesillas, Treaty of, 14–15

Totsuka Seikai, 129, 162

Toyotomi Hideyoshi: treatment of medical missionaries in Japan, 14, 16

Udagawa Genshin: father of pharmacology in Japan, 100; helped compile Dutch-Japanese diction-

THE JOHNS HOPKINS PRESS

Designed by Arlene J. Sheer

Composed in Monotype Baskerville text and display
by Baltimore Type and Composition Corporation

Printed on 60-lb. Warren 1854
by The Colonial Press, Inc.

Bound in Holliston Roxite
by The Colonial Press, Inc.